Practical
Bovine & Ovine
Diagnosis & Treatment
in Late Qing Imperial China

A Handbook of Veterinary Herbology for Cattle & Sheep

Transcribed & Translated from an Original French & Chinese Text of 1863

Dr. Colin B. Lessell

MMXX

First Published 2020
Samphire Press
Suthsæxe, England

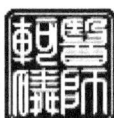

Other books on Chinese topics by the same author:

Bibliotheca Medica de Asia Orientali 1473-1900

*A New Translation of Abel-Rémusat's
Classical Chinese Grammar 1822 & 1857*

Menu Chinese Made Easy

Jesuit Pharmacy in 17th Century China

*A Catalogue of Chinese Mineral Drugs :
current or obsolete, curious or bizarre,
therapeutic or toxic*

Tongue Diagnosis in 17th Century China

*Practical Equine Diagnosis & Treatment
in Late Qing Imperial China*

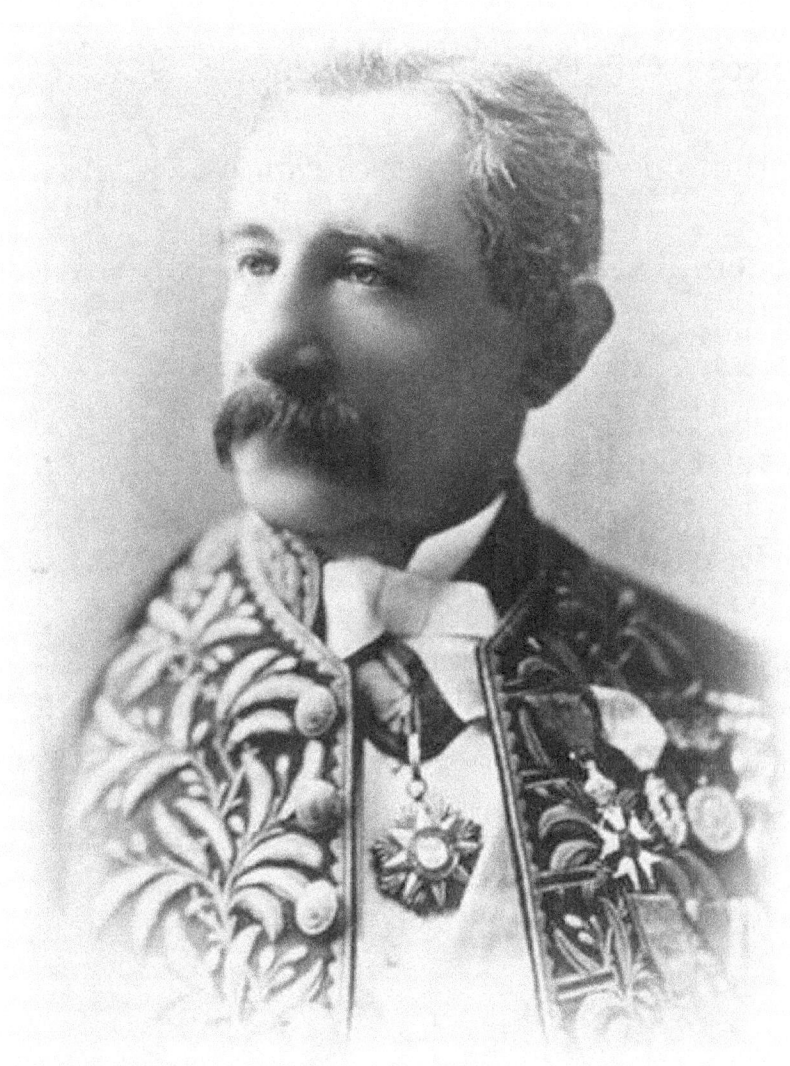

Claude Philibert Dabry de Thiersant c. 1878

CONTENTS

LA MÉDECINE

CHEZ

LES CHINOIS

PAR

Le capitaine P. DABRY

CONSUL DE FRANCE EN CHINE, CHEVALIER DE LA LÉGION D'HONNEUR,
MEMBRE DE LA SOCIÉTÉ ASIATIQUE DE PARIS.

OUVRAGE CORRIGÉ ET PRÉCÉDÉ D'UNE PRÉFACE

PAR

M. J. Léon SOUBEIRAN

DOCTEUR EN MÉDECINE, DOCTEUR ÈS SCIENCES, PROFESSEUR AGRÉGÉ À L'ÉCOLE DE PHARMACIE.

———

ORNÉ DE PLANCHES ANATOMIQUES.

PARIS

HENRI PLON, IMPRIMEUR ÉDITEUR,
RUE GARANCIÈRE, 8.

1863

Title Page of *La médecine chez les chinois* 1863

INTRODUCTION

This monograph is a full transcription and translation of an account by Captain P. Dabry in 1863, being the *only* significant European description of Chinese bovine & ovine medicine published before modern times. As such, it is of considerable historical importance to those interested in, or involved with, TCVM (Traditional Chinese Veterinary Medicine) as it applies to livestock. Beyond that, with regards to decisions of safety and efficacy, I must emphasise that these are not the province of the current translator, but must rest firmly and exclusively on the shoulders of my readers. Having thus absolved myself of this responsibility, let us now begin by considering the relevant background of the original author.

Claude Philibert Dabry (1826-1898) began his career in the French navy (see Frontispiece). In 1856, he was promoted to the rank of captain. From 1856 to 1862, he was stationed as government commissioner in Tianjin and the Zhoushan Islands. In 1863, he was entrusted with the French consulate in Hankou, a position which he held until 1868. In 1868, he combined his father's name with his mother's, and thereafter called himself Dabry de Thiersant. He then occupied various diplomatic functions in the consulates of Shanghai (1868-1869) and Guangzhou (1869-1871).

Being fully conversant with spoken and written Chinese, and having a profound interest in the Chinese style of both human and veterinary medicine, up to 1863 (and perhaps beyond), he set about translating various original works on these subjects. With regard to the availability of livestock source books in his day, you are recommended to consult the list of such provided at the end of the current monograph. Moreover, it is not unreasonable to assume that he also sought instruction and guidance from local practitioners. The content of the text certainly suggests the use of multiple anonymous sources.

In 1863, having spent some seven years in China, his extensive work of 580 pages, *La médecine chez les chinois* (Medicine amongst the Chinese), was published in Paris, under his original name, *Le capitaine P. Dabry*, and (those were the days) at the expense of the French government. (Title Page reproduced on p. 5.) Remarkably, it covered every aspect, including traditional theory, pulse diagnosis, acupuncture and medicinal prescriptions; all in rather tiny print. In its production, not being a doctor of medicine himself, he had employed to advantage the assistance of Dr. Jean Léon Soubeiran M.D. (1827-1892), professor at the Montpellier School of Pharmacy in France.

However, the only part of the book with which we are here concerned is that entitled *Maladies des bœufs et des moutons* (Diseases of cattle and sheep), under the general title *Art vétérinaire* (Veterinary science), and this has been fully transcribed (with a few well-marked typographical corrections) within the current monograph, with all such transcribed passages being highlighted in grey. The bulk of the treatments are medicinal (largely herbal), with the occasional brief mention of other techniques, including phlebotomy (bleeding) and nutrition. It essentially constitutes a handbook of livestock herbology in its own right. (The section of *Art vétérinaire* concerning equine diseases, *Maladies des cheveax,* has been dealt with in a previous volume of mine: *Practical equine diagnosis & treatment in late Qing imperial China.*)

Maladies des bœufs et des moutons is divided into 67 sections of named diseases or syndromes, each with its own heading, covering over 60 different disorders of livestock. Though they are unnumbered in the original text, for the purpose of reference, I have divided them into individually enumerated subsections, with the initial untranslated heading subsection boxed, with highlighting in grey. For clarity, this is always found at the top of a page. As might be expected, the basic text is in straightforward French, including the symptomatic pictures (apart from the occasional romanized Chinese name for a disease), and this has been reliably translated into English. However, when we come to the treatment subsections, the names of the medications (herbs, minerals and the odd animal substance) are nearly all in romanized Chinese.

As with the rest of the book, there are no Chinese characters to guide us, nor indeed any indication of syllabic tone (so important in deciphering a language with a limited syllabic repertoire). Moreover, the romanization is of a non-standard (pre-Wade-Giles) type, with decided French and dialectal influences (e.g. *choui* for *shui*, and *hiang* for *xiang*), and a modicum of inconsistency. Despite these problems, since the range of possible matches is generally quite limited, translation of the names of medications into modern Pinyin, Chinese characters (including simplified forms), Latin or chemical titles, and common English names (where possible) has been carried out with a high degree of accuracy and thus reliability.

The same, however, cannot be said of most of the headings of the sections which inform us of the *names* of the diseases or syndromes. Consistent with Dabry's reverence for the concepts of TCM (Traditional Chinese Medicine), they mainly include terminology peculiar to this ancient system. (Helpfully, but only in *Maladies des cheveaux,* he does give us bracketed French clues to the meaning of 49 of its section headings; and these have also been found useful in the current translation.) Some individual syllables are indeed easily identified (e.g. *fong* for pathogenic wind), but the lack of tone markings on more common syllables, plus the degree of ellipsis (exclusion of words, especially prepositions), so typical of Classical Chinese, can lead to some confusion over the exact meaning of a phrase. Another pitfall is to fail to realise that syllables obviously referring to internal organs (such as *liver* or *lung*) also often refer to the channel or meridian system with which they are associated. Similar problems can also arise occasionally in the translation of the name of a particular compound prescription. However, these matters in no way influence the correct identification of a disorder by means of its symptomatic picture or indeed the composition of its supposed appropriate therapy; and thus the implied practicality of the text is ensured.

A final point to be made concerns the weights used for medicinal substances in the text. With the exception of the *livre* (about 1lb/500g), they all are conveniently in *grams*. The rather strange quantities of 3.68g, 7.36g and 11.04g found in the text are concerned with equivalence to the Chinese pharmaceutical weight system, as would be found in old literature, based upon the *qián* 錢. Thus:

1 *qián* = 3.68g
2 *qián* = 2 x 3.68g = 7.36g
3 *qián* = 3 x 3.68g = 11.04g

Such precision was almost certainly provided by Professor Soubeiran, with whom Dabry de Thiersant (as he then became) later collaborated to publish *La matière médicale chez les chinois* (Materia medica amongst the Chinese) in 1874. Whilst of some general interest, it is a book which has been of only minimal assistance to the current translation.

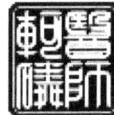

REFERENCES

Bensky, D. ; Clavey, S. ; Stöger, E. ; Gamble, A. (2004) *Chinese herbal medicine : materia medica.* 3rd edn. Seattle: Eastland Press.

Cisheng, Jiang *et al* (1991) *A Chinese-English dictionary of traditional Chinese veterinary medicine.* China: Agricultural Publishing House.

Dabry, P. ; Soubeiran, J.L. (1863) *La médecine chez les chinois.* Paris: Henri Plon.

Fèvre, F. ; Métailé, G. (2005) *Dictionnaire Ricci des plantes de Chine.* Paris: Ricci Cerf.

Giles, H.A (1892) *A Chinese-English dictionary.* London: Quaritch. Shanghai, Hongkong, Yokohama, Singapore: Kelly & Walsh.

Lessell, C.B. (2016) *Bibliotheca medica de Asia orientali 1473-1900.* 6th edn. CD. Suthsaexe, England: Samphire Press.

Lessell, C.B. (2018) *A catalogue of Chinese mineral drugs.* Suthsaexe, England: Samphire Press.

Lessell, C.B. (2018) *Jesuit pharmacy in 17th century China.* Suthsaexe, England: Samphire Press.

Lessell, C.B. (2019) *Practical equine diagnosis & treatment in late Qing imperial China..* Suthsaexe, England: Samphire Press.

Scheid, V. ; Bensky, D. ; Ellis, A. ; Barolet, R. (2015) *Chinese herbal medicine : formulas & strategies.* Portable 2nd edn. Seattle (WA): Eastland Press.

Smith, F.P. (1871) *Contributions towards the materia medica & natural history of China.* London: Trübner.

Song, Dalu ; Xie, Huisheng ; et al. (2012) *Annotated Yuan Heng's classical collection on the treatment of equine diseases.* Beijing: China Agriculture Press.

Soubeiran, J.L. ; Dabry de Thiersant [C.P.] (1874) *La matière médicale chez les chinois.* Paris: Masson.

Stuart, Revd. G.A. ; Smith, F.P. (1911) *Chinese materia medica : vegetable kingdom.* Shanghai: American Presbyterian Press.

Wiseman, N. (1995) *Dictionary of Chinese medicine* : English-Chinese, Chinese-English. Hunan: Hunan Science Technology Press.

Xie, Huisheng ; Preast, V. (2010) *Xie's Chinese veterinary herbology.* Ames (IA): Wiley-Blackwell.

MALADIES DES BŒUFS ET DES MOUTONS.

DISEASES OF CATTLE & SHEEP.

§ **Fr 1.1**   *Fey-oey.*

L'animal ne veut pas travailler; inappétence; il se couche, souffle par les naseaux, tête levée vers le ciel, yeux larmoyants; mouvements des mâchoires, oppression.

§ **Tr 1.1**   *fèi wèi*
                                              肺胃
                                              lung & stomach

The animal does not want to work; loss of appetite; he lies down, puffing throgh the nostrils, his head raised to the sky, his eyes watering; jaw movements, breathlessness.

Fr 1.2 Lui donner *hing-jin-san. – Hing-jin, tchin-tchou, ngo-kiao, me-men-tong, pe-tsee, hoa-lo, nieou-pang-tsee, kie-keng* (11^g chacun); réduire en poudre; alun (36^g), *kiang-houang* (36^g); faire bouillir; lui donner trois ou quatre fois.

Tr 1.2 *Give it :- **xìng rén săn** 杏仁散 Apricot Kernel Powder*:
- *hing-jin* = **xìng rén** 杏仁 Prunus spp. seed/kernel. Apricot.
- *tchin-tchou* = **jīn zhú** 1. 篁竹 Bamboo (S. China sp.) leaf/root. 2. 金竹 Phyllostachys sulphurea bamboo shavings.
- *ngo-kiao* = **ē jiāo** 阿膠 (阿胶) Ass/donkey-hide gelatin/glue.
- *me-men-tong* = **mài mén dōng** 麥門冬 (麦门冬) Ophiopogon japonicus tuber. Ophiopogon. Mondo grass.
- *pe-tsee* = **bái zhǐ** 白芷 Angelica dahurica root. Dahurican angelica.
- *hoa-lo* = **guā lóu** 瓜蔞 (瓜蒌) Trichosanthes kirilowii/ rosthornii fruit. Chinese cucumber.

- *nieou-pang-tsee* = ***niú bàng zǐ*** 牛蒡子 Arctium lappa fruit. Great burdock.
- *kie-keng* = ***jié gěng*** 桔梗 Platycodon grandiflorus root. Balloon flower.

11g of each of the above.

Reduce to a powder; add:

- alun = ***alum.***   *36g.*
- *kiang-houang* = ***jiāng húang*** 薑黃（姜黃）Curcuma spp. root. *Inc.* turmeric.   *36g.*

- ***Boil.***

Give three or four times.

§ **Fr 2.1** *Choui-ho-tan.*

L'animal se couche, tourne la tête; mouvements des mâchoires; par la bouche coulent des mucosités jaunes; oreilles froides, agitation, yeux larmoyants; maladie grave.

§ **Tr 2.1** *shuǐ hé dǎn*
水合膽(水合胆)
water [= kidney] combined with gallbladder

The animal lies down, turns its head; jaw movements; yellow mucus flows from the mouth; cold ears, agitation, watery eyes; a serious illness.

Fr 2.2 *Sse-tchuen-san. – Houei-hiang, houei-hoa, tsang-chou, pe-tchou* (2^g ½); réduire en poudre; sel (36^g), *seng-kiang* (36^g); faire bouillir.

Tr 2.2 *sì chuān sǎn* 四川散 *Sichuan Powder*:

- *houei-hiang* = **huí xiāng** 茴香 Foeniculum vulgare fruit. Fennel.
- *houei-hoa* = **huǐ huā** 檓花 Zanthoxylum bungeanum. pericarp. Sichuan pepper.
- *tsang-chou* = **cháng chǔ** 萇楚(苌楚) Actinidia chinensis/rufa fruit. A type of kiwi fruit.
- *pe-tchou* = **bái chǒu** 白丑 Pharbitis spp. seed. Morning glory.

2.5 g. [of each].

Reduce to a powder.

Add:

- sel = ***salt.***   *36g.*
- *seng-kiang* = ***shēng jiāng*** 生薑 (生姜) Zingiber officinalis fresh rhizome. Ginger.   *36g.*

- ***Boil.***

§ **Fr 3.1**   *Han-hoang-ping.*

L'animal se couche; tête levée, queue remuant toujours; quelquefois l'animal se lève comme un furieux et court de tous côtés; langue et lèvres noires; affection très-grave.

§ **Tr 3.1**   *gān huáng bìng*
肝黃病（肝黄病）
yellow liver disease

The animal lies down; head raised, tail always swishing; sometimes the animal rises as though enraged and runs about everywhere; tongue and lips black; a very grave affection.

Fr 3.2 Remède : *Tien-tchou-hoang-tsin. — Yuen-seng, tien-tchou-hoang, tcho-kien-tsee, tsin-siang-tsee, che-kiue-ming, nieou-pang-tsee, kan-tsao. ta-hoang, pan-tchou-suen* (7^g,36), *po-siao* (150^g), *tsee-tsiao* (150^g); faire bouillir.

Tr 3.2 Remedy :- ***tiān zhú huáng zhèn*** 天竺黃鎮（天竺黄镇）
Tabasheer Tranquilizer:
- *yuen-seng* = ***yuán shēn*** 元參（元参）Scrophularia ningpoensis root. Ningpo figwort
- *tien-tchou-hoang* = ***tiān zhú huáng*** 天竺黃（天竺黄）Tabasheer. Siliceous secretions of bamboo.
- *tcho-kien-tsee* = ***chē qián zī*** 車前子（车前子）Plantago spp. seed. Plantago.
- *tsin-siang-tsee* = ***qīng xiāng zǐ*** 青香子 Celosia argentea seed. Celosia.
- *che-kiue-ming* = ***shí jué míng*** 石決明（石决明）Haliotis spp. shell. Abalone.

- *nieou-pang-tsee* = **niú bàng zǐ** 牛蒡子 Arctium lappa fruit. Great burdock.
- *kan-tsao* = **gān cǎo** 甘草（甘艸）Glycyrrhiza spp. root. Licorice. Liquorice.
- *ta-hoang* = **dà huáng** 大黃（大黄）Rheum spp. root/rhizome. Rhubarb.
- *pan-tchou-suen* = 1. **bān jiū zhān** 斑鳩佔（斑鸠佔）Premna puberula root/leaf. 2. **bān jiū zhàn** 斑鳩站（斑鸠站）Premna ligustroides fructification/root/leaf.

  7.36g [of each].

- *po-siao* = **pǔ xiāo** 朴消 Glauber's salt. Mirabilite.

  150g.

- *tsee-tsiao* = **zhǐ qiào** 枳殼（枳壳）Citrus aurantium fruit. Bitter orange. *150g.*

- **Boil.**

§ **Fr 4.1**   *Fey-hoang-ping.*

Yeux égarés; l'animal frappe le mur avec ses cornes, oppression, crampes; il se couche.

§ **Tr 4.1**   *fèi huáng bìng*
肺黄病(肺黄病)
yellow lung disease

Wild eyes; the animal strikes the wall with its horns, breathlessness, cramps; it lies down.

Fr 4.2 Traitement : *Tsang-pou-san. — Tsang-pou, pe-tche, tche-mou, ta-hoang, pe-mou, ouen-ho, kan-tsao, hoa-lo-jin* (4ᵍ), *pe-fan* (1 livre), miel (150ᵍ); faire bouillir; donner quatre ou cinq fois.

Tr 4.2 Treatment :- ***chāng pú sǎn*** 菖蒲散 *Acorus Powder*:
- *tsang-pou* = ***chāng pú*** 菖蒲 Acorus calamus rhizome. Sweetflag.
- *pe-tche* = ***bái chǒu*** 白丑 Pharbitis spp. seed. Morning glory.
- *tche-mou* = ***zhī mǔ*** 知母 Anemarrhena asphodeloides rhizome. Anemarrhena.
- *ta-hoang* = ***dà huáng*** 大黄(大黄) Rheum spp. root/rhizome. Rhubarb.
- *pe-mou* = ***bèi mǔ*** 貝母(贝母) Fritillaria spp. bulb. Fritillary.
- *ouen-ho* = ***yuán hú*** 元胡 Corydalis yanhusuo rhizome. Corydalis.
- *kan-tsao* = ***gān cǎo*** 甘草(甘艹) Glycyrrhiza spp. root. Licorice. Liquorice.

- *hoa-lo-jin* = **guā lóu rén** 瓜蔞仁（瓜蒌仁）Trichosanthes kirilowii/rosthornii seed. Chinese cucumber.

  4g [of each].

- *pe-fan* = **bái fán** 白礬（白矾）Alum. *about 1 lb/500g.*
- miel = **honey.** *150g.*

- **Boil.**

Give four or five times.

§ **Fr 5.1**   *Sin-fong-hoang-ping.*

Oppression, écume autour de la bouche, yeux enflés, boutons ronds ou de forme ovoide sur le corps, mouvements des mâchoires et de la tête.

§ **Tr 5.1**   *xīn fēng huáng bìng*
心風黃病（心风黄病）
yellow heart wind disease

Breathlessness, froth around the mouth, swollen eyes, round or ovoid papules on the body, movements of the jaw and head.

Fr 5.2 Traitement : *Jin-seng-san. — Jin-seng, fou-ling, hoang-pe, yu-kin, ching-ma, tsin-tan, kan-tsao, ping-lang-ken* (7^g,36); réduire en poudre; *seng-kiang* (120^g); faire bouillir.

Tr 5.2   Treatment :- *rén shēn sǎn* 人參散（人参散）*Ginseng Powder*:

- *jin-seng* = *rén shēn* 人參（人参）Panax ginseng root. Ginseng.
- *fou-ling* = *fú líng* 茯苓 Poria cocos. Poria. China root.
- *hoang-pe* = *huáng bǎi* 黃柏（黄柏）Phellodendron spp. bark. Amur cork tree.
- *yu-kin* = *yù jīn* 鬱金（郁金）Curcuma spp. root. *Inc.* turmeric.
- *ching-ma* = *qǐng má* 苘麻 Abutilon theophrasti seed. Chingma abutilon. Chinese jute. Indian mallow.
- *tsin-tan* = *qīng tán* 青檀 Dalbergia hupeana bark/root-bark.
- *kan-tsao* = *gān cǎo* 甘草（甘艹）Glycyrrhiza spp. root.

- *ping-lang-ken* = **bīng láng rén** 檳榔仁（槟榔仁）Areca catechu nut kernel. Betel.

  7.36g [of each].

  Reduce to a powder.

- *seng-kiang* = **shēng jiāng** 生薑（生姜）Zingiber officinalis fresh rhizome. Ginger. *120g.*

- **Boil.**

> **§ Fr 6.1**   *Hoang-tien-cheou-ping.*
>
> Oppression, maigreur; quelquefois subitement tout le corps enflé; l'animal n'aime pas à travailler; urine rouge.

§ Tr 6.1   *huáng diàn shòu bìng*
黃潭瘦病（黄潭瘦病）
yellow oedema wasting disease

Breathlessness, thinness; sometimes suddenly all the body becomes swollen; the animal does not like to work; red urine.

Fr 6.2 Traitement : *Ou-kin-san. — Mo-yo, chao-yo, ki-ling-kiai, hoang-pe, tsien-lieou, tsou-yu, ly-kou-py, kan-tsao, ta-houang, kou-hoang-lien* (7^g,36), faire bouillir.

Tr 6.2 Treatment :- ***wǔ jīng sǎn*** 五經散（五经散）*Five Channels Powder*:

- *mo-yo* = ***mò yào*** 沒藥（沒药） Myrrh.
- *chao-yo* = ***sháo yào*** 芍藥（芍药） Paeonia spp. rubra root. Red peony root.
- *ki-ling-kiai* = ***qí lín jié*** 麒麟竭 Daemonorops draco resin. Dragon's blood.
- *hoang-pe* = ***huáng bǎi*** 黃柏（黄柏） Phellodendron spp. bark. Amur cork tree.
- *tsien-lieou* = ***chēng liǔ*** 檉柳（柽柳） Tamarix chinensis twig & leaf. Tamarisk.
- *tsou-yu* = ***zhú yóu*** 竹油 Bamboo sap.
- *ly-kou-py* = ***lì shù pí*** 栗樹皮（栗树皮） Castanea mollissima bark. Chinese chestnut.

- *kan-tsao* = **gān cǎo** 甘草（甘艸）Glycyrrhiza spp. root. Licorice. Liquorice.
- *ta-houang* = **dà huáng** 大黃（大黄）Rheum spp. root/rhizome. Rhubarb.
- *kou-hoang-lien* = **chǎo huáng lián** 炒黃連（炒黄连）Coptis spp. dry-fried rhizome. Goldthread.

7.36g [of each].

- ***Boil.***

§ **Fr 7.1** *Sin-hoang-ping.*

L'animal court comme un furieux; yeux fixes, mouvements de la queue, chaleur dans le corps, souffle brûlant.

§ **Tr 7.1** *xīn huáng bìng*
心黃病(心黃病)
yellow heart disease

The animal runs about as though enraged; fixed eyes, tail swishing, hot body, very hot breath.

Fr 7.2 Traitement : *Kin-tsin-san. – Jin-seng, fou-ling, tsin-tay, ta-hoang, ping-lang, kan-tsao, tsee-tsee* (7^g,36 chacun); réduire en poudre; miel (180^g); eau chaude.

Tr 7.2 Treatment :- ***rén qīng săn*** 人青散 *Ginseng & Indigo Powder*:
- *jin-seng* = ***rén shēn*** 人參(人参) Panax ginseng root. Ginseng.
- *fou-ling* = ***fú líng*** 茯苓 Poria cocos. Poria. China root.
- *tsin-tay* = ***qīng dài*** 青黛 Indigo naturalis. Indigo.
- *ta-hoang* = ***dà huáng*** 大黃(大黄) Rheum spp. root/rhizome. Rhubarb.
- *ping-lang* = ***bīng láng*** 檳榔(槟榔) Areca catechu nut. Betel.
- *kan-tsao* = ***gān căo*** 甘草(甘艹) Glycyrrhiza spp. root. Licorice. Liquorice.

- *tsee-tsee* = **zhī zǐ** 梔子（栀子） Gardenia jasminoides fruit. Cape jasmine.

7.36g of each of the above.

Reduce to a powder.

- miel = **honey.**   *180g.*
- **hot water.**

[Compare ℞ in **52.2** below.]

> **§ Fr 8.1**   *Lao-tchong-hoang.*
>
> Se couche sur le dos.

§ Tr 8.1   *láo zhōng huáng*
                                 勞中黃 (劳中黄)
                                 yellow centre taxation

Lies down on its back.

Fr 8.2   Traitement : *Ting-fong-san. — Tien-tchou-hoang, fang-fong, jin-seng, tchuen-kio, seng-ty, tsee-seng, tien-ma, ma-hoang, pe-ky-ly, kan-tsao, fou-tsee* (7^g,36 chacun); *miel* (72^g); faire bouillir.

Tr 8.2   Treatment :- ***dìng fēng sǎn*** 定風散 (定风散) *Settle Wind Powder*:
- *tien-tchou-hoang* = ***tiān zhú huáng*** 天竺黃 (天竺黄) Tabasheer. Siliceous secretions of bamboo.
- *fang-fong* = ***fáng fēng*** 防風 (防风) Saposhnikovia divaricata root. Saposhnikovia.
- *jin-seng* = ***rén shēn*** 人參 (人参) Panax ginseng root. Ginseng.
- *tchuen-kio* = ***chuān jiāo*** 川椒 Zanthoxylum bungeanum pericarp. Sichuan pepper.
- *seng-ty* = ***shēng dì*** 生地 Rehmannia glutinosa root. Chinese foxglove.
- *tsee-seng* = ***zǐ shēn*** 紫參 (紫参) Polygonum bistorta rhizome. Bistort.
- *tien-ma* = ***tiān má*** 天麻 Gastrodia elata rhizome. Gastrodia.
- *ma-hoang* = ***má huáng*** 麻黃 (麻黄) Ephedra spp. leaf/stem. Ephedra.

- *pe-ky-ly* = **bái jí lí** 白蒺藜 Tribulus terrestris fruit. Caltrop. Puncture vine.
- *kan-tsao* = **gān căo** 甘草（甘艸）Glycyrrhiza spp. root. Licorice. Liquorice.
- *fou-tsee* = **fù zǐ** 附子 Aconitum carmichaeli prepared accessory root. Sichuan aconite.

7.36g of each of the above.

- miel = **honey.**   *72g.*

- **Boil.**

§ **Fr 9.1** *Tsao-chong-pi.*

Oppression, souffle bruyant, borborygmes continuels, poils hérissés, diarrhée, mouvements des mâchoires,; langue rouge.

§ **Tr 9.1** *căo qióng pi*
草窮脾（草穷脾）
grass exhaustion spleen

Breathlessness, continual noisy bowel sounds, hair stands on end, diarrhoea, jaw movements; red tongue.

Fr 9.2 *Tchuen-chang-san. — Kien-lieou, ta-hoang, kan-soui, pe-ky, hoang-tsin, hoa-che, hoang-kin* (7ᵍ,36); réduire en poudre; *po-siao* (100ᵍ); faire bouillir; graisse de cochon.

Tr 9.2 *chuāng shāng săn* 創傷散（创伤散） *Trauma Powder*:
- *kien-lieou* = *jiàn [yè] liŭ* 箭［葉］蓼（箭［叶］蓼）Polygonum sieboldii seed/entire. Smartweed.
- *ta-hoang* = *dà huáng* 大黃（大黄）Rheum spp. root/rhizome. Rhubarb.
- *kan-soui* = *gān suì* 甘遂 Euphorbia kansui root. Kan-sui.
- *pe-ky* = *bái jí* 白及 Bletilla striata rhizome. Bletilla.
- *hoang-tsin* = *huáng qín* 黃芩（黄芩）Scutellaria baicalensis root. Baical skullcap.
- *hoa-che* = *huá shí* 滑石 Talcum.
- *hoang-kin* = *huáng jīng* 黃精（黄精）Polygonatum spp. rhizome. Siberian Solomon's seal.

7.36g [of each].

Reduce to a powder.

- *po-siao* = **pǔ xiāo** 朴消 Glauber's salt. Mirabilite.   *100g*

- **Boil**.

- [*Add* :-] graisse de cochon = **lard**.

---

§ **Fr 10.1**   *Choui-teou-fong.*

Tête enflée, sueur sur tout le corps, délire, yeux fixe.

---

§ **Tr 10.1**   *shuǐ tóu fẽng*
水頭風（水头风）
water & wind in head

Head swollen, sweat all over his body, delirium, eyes fixed.

Fr 10.2 Traitement : *Chin-chan-san.* – *Pi-choang* (2^g), *pong-cha* (1^g,50), *hoang-tang,* réduire en poudre (2^g), miel (36^g), *jou-hiang, me-tong* (36^g).

Tr 10.2 Treatment :- **shèn shāng sǎn** 腎傷散（肾伤散）*Kidney Damage Powder*:

- *pi-choang* = **pī shuāng** 砒霜 Sublimed arsenic.   *2g.*

- *pong-cha* = **péng shā** 硼砂 Borax.   *1.5g.*

- *hoang-tang* = **huáng dān** 黃丹（黄丹）Massicot. Yellow lead oxide.   *2g.*

                         Reduce to a powder.

- miel = **honey.**   *36g.*

- *jou-hiang* = **rù xiāng** 乳香 Olibanum. Frankincense.   *[36g].*

- *me-tong* = **mài dōng** 麥冬（麦冬）Ophiopogon japonicus tuber. Ophiopogon. Mondo grass.   *36g.*

> **§ Fr 11.1** *Tsi-ho-tchuen.*
>
> Râle dans la gorge, poitrail enflé, inappétence, ventre enflé, mouvements des mâchoires.

§ Tr 11.1 *qī hé chuāng*
凄合創（凄合创）
intense cold trauma

Rattling in throat, chest swollen, lack of appetite, swollen belly, jaw movements.

Fr 11.2 Traitement : saigner; *pe-fan-san. — Pe-fan, pe-mou, hoang-lien, pe-tsee, yu-kin, hoang-tsin, ta-hoang, kan-tsao, ting-ly* (7^g,36); poudre; miel (150^g), eau chaude.

Tr 11.2 Treatment :- bleed; ***bái fán săn*** 白礬散（白矾散）*Alum Powder*:

- *pe-fan* = ***bái fán*** 白礬（白矾）Alum.
- *pe-mou* = ***bèi mŭ*** 貝母（贝母）Fritillaria spp. bulb. Fritillary.
- *hoang-lien* = ***huáng lián*** 黃連（黄连）Coptis spp. rhizome. Goldthread.
- *pe-tsee* = ***bái zhĭ*** 白芷 Angelica dahurica root. Dahurican angelica.
- *yu-kin* = ***yù jīn*** 鬱金（郁金）Curcuma spp. root. *Inc.* turmeric.
- *hoang-tsin* = ***huáng qín*** 黃芩（黄芩）Scutellaria baicalensis root. Baical skullcap.
- *ta-hoang* = ***dà huáng*** 大黃（大黄）Rheum spp. root/rhizome.
- *kan-tsao* = ***gān căo*** 甘草（甘艸）Glycyrrhiza spp. root.

31

- *ting-ly* = **tíng lì [zǐ]** 葶藶［子］（葶苈［子］）Lepidium apetalum/ Descurainia sophia/Rorippa montana seed. Tingli.

  7.36g [of each].

  Reduce to a powder.

- miel = **honey.**   *150g.*
- **hot water.**

§ **Fr 12.1**   *Nieou-hiue-ping.*

Inappétence, constipation, délire; corps froid, urine sanguino-lente, fièvre.

§ **Tr 12.1**   *niú xuè bìng*
牛血病
cow's bleeding disorder

Lack of appetite, constipation, delirium; cold body, urine tinged with blood, fever.

Fr 12.2 Traitement : *Tang-kouei-san.* – ***[Tang-kouei,*]*** *Mo-yo, cho-yo, sy-sin, kouei-hiang, pe-tchou, kouei-hoa, jo-kouei* (7^g,36); réduire en poudre; *seng-kiang* (36^g), sel (150^g); faire bouillir.

Tr 12.2   Treatment :- ***dāng guī sǎn*** 當歸散（当归散）*Angelica Powder*:

- *[tang-kouei*]* = ***dāng guī*** 當歸（当归）Angelica sinensis root. Chinese angelica.   *omitted in the original in error
- *mo-yo* = ***mò yào*** 沒藥（沒药）Myrrh.
- *cho-yo* = ***sháo yào*** 芍藥（芍药）Paeonia spp. rubra root. Red peony root.
- *sy-sin* = ***xì xīn*** 細辛（细辛）Asarum spp. root/rhizome. Chinese wild ginger.
- *kouei-hiang* = ***guǐ jiàn*** 鬼箭 Euonymus alatus 'wings'/twigs. Spindle tree.
- *pe-tchou* = ***bái chǒu*** 白丑 Pharbitis spp. seed. Morning glory.
- *kouei-hoa* = ***guì huā*** 桂花 Osmanthus fragrans flower. Sweet osmanthus.

- *jo-kouei* = **ròu guì** 肉桂 Cinnamomum cassia inner bark. Saigon cinnamon.

  7.36g [of each].

  Reduce to a powder.

- *seng-kiang* = **shēng jiāng** 生薑(生姜) Zingiber officinalis fresh rhizome. Ginger.   *36g.*
- sel = **salt.**   *150g.*

- **Boil.**

§ **Fr 13.1**   *Kan-tchang-fang.*

L'animal couche et se lève, yeux fixes; quelquefois il court comme un furieux; ventre enflé, il remue la tête, langue et lèvres bleues.

§ **Tr 13.1**   *gān cháng fāng*
乾腸方（干肠方）
dry intestine remedy

The animal lies down & gets up; sometimes it runs around as though it were mad; bloated belly, it shakes its head, the tongue and lips blue.

Fr 13.2 Traitement : *Han-siao-fa. — Hoang-tsin, tsin-hiang-tsee, che-kiue-ming, tsao-kiue-ming, che-kao, lang-tan-tsao, yuen-kin-che, nieou-pang-tsee, po-siao* (7ᵍ,36), miel (150ᵍ), eau chaude.

Tr 13.2 Treatment :- ***gān xiāo fā*** 肝消伐 *Liver Disperser & Queller*:

- *hoang-tsin* = ***huáng qín*** 黃芩（黄芩） Scutellaria baicalensis root. Baical skullcap.
- *tsin-hiang-tsee* = ***qīng xiāng zǐ*** 青香子 Celosia argentea seed. Celosia.
- *che-kiue-ming* = ***shí jué míng*** 石決明（石决明） Haliotis spp. shell. Abalone.
- *tsao-kiue-ming* = ***cǎo jué míng*** 草決明 Cassia spp. seed. Foetid cassia.
- *che-kao* = ***shí gāo*** 石膏 Crystalline gypsum.
- *lang-tan-tsao* = ***làng dàng cǎo*** 茛菪艸（茛菪草） Hyoscyamus niger root. Henbane.

- *yuen-kin-che* = **yuán qín qiē** 元芩切 Scutellaria baicalensis root slices. Baical skullcap.
- *nieou-pang-tsee* = **niú bàng zǐ** 牛蒡子 Arctium lappa fruit. Great burdock.
- *po-siao* = **pǔ xiāo** 樸消（朴消）Glauber's salt.

7.36g [of each].

- miel = **honey.**   *150g.*
- **hot water.**

§ **Fr 14.1** *Choui-tsao-tchang.*

Inappétence, écume autour de la bouche, ventre enflé, langue pendante, écoulement de mucosités.

§ **Tr 14.1** *shuĭ căo cháng*
水艸腸(水草腸)
water & grass intestines

Lack of appetite, froth around the mouth, swollen belly, tongue hanging out, flow of mucus,

Fr 14.2 Traitement : *Ta-ky-san.* — *Ta-ky, hoa-che, kan-soui, kien-lieou, hoang-tsin, pa-teou, ta-hoang* (7ᵍ,36); *po-siao* (36ᵍ); faire bouillir.

Tr 14.2 Treatment :- ***dà jĭ săn*** 大戟散 *Euphorbia* Powder*:

- *Ta-ky* = ***dà jĭ*** 大戟 Euphorbia pekinensis root*. Peking spurge. [*This traditional root, in view of its higher level of toxicity, is now usually replaced with ***hóng dà jĭ*** 紅大戟(红大戟) Knoxia valerianoides root. Knoxia.]
- *hoa-che* = ***huá shí*** 滑石 Talcum.
- *kan-soui* = ***gān suì*** 甘遂 Euphorbia kansui root. Kan-sui.
- *kien-lieou* = ***jiàn [yè] liŭ*** 箭[葉]蓼(箭[叶]蓼) Polygonum sieboldii seed/entire. Smartweed.
- *hoang-tsin* = ***huáng qín*** 黃芩(黄芩) Scutellaria baicalensis root. Baical skullcap.
- *pa-teou* = ***bā dòu*** 巴豆 Croton tiglium fruit. Croton.

- *ta-hoang* = **dà huáng** 大黃（大黃）Rheum spp. root/rhizome. Rhubarb.

  7.36g [of each].

- *po-siao* = **pǔ xiāo** 朴消 Glauber's salt. Mirabilite. *36g.*

- **Boil.**

> **§ Fr 15.1**   *Pe-ye-kan.*
>
> Maigreur, l'animal ne veut pas travailler; tête basse, mouvements des machoires; des mucosités coulent par la bouche.

§ Tr 15.1   *bǎi yè gān*
百葉乾(百叶干)
dry stomach

Thinness, the animal does not want to work; low head, jaw movements; mucus flows from the mouth.

Fr 15.2 Traitement : *Tchou-tche-san. — Pe-tsee, ty-yu-py, hoa-che, tsien-lieou, kan-tsao, jou-kouei, kan-sui, ta-ky, sin-chou-tsee* (7^g,36); réduire en poudre; graisse de cochon (1/2 livre), miel (72^g), eau chaude.

Tr 15.2 Treatment :- *zhōu chē sǎn* 舟車散(舟车散)*Boats & Carts Powder*:

- *pe-tsee* = *bái zhǐ* 白芷 Angelica dahurica root. Dahurican angelica.
- *ty-yu-py* = *dì yú pí* 地榆皮 Sanguisorba officinalis root bark. Burnet-bloodwort.
- *hoa-che* = *huá shí* 滑石 Talcum.
- *tsien-lieou* = *chēng liǔ* 檉柳(柽柳) Tamarix chinensis twig & leaf. Tamarisk.
- *kan-tsao* = *gān cǎo* 甘草(甘艸) Glycyrrhiza spp. root. Licorice. Liquorice.
- *jou-kouei* = *ròu guì* 肉桂 Cinnamomum cassia inner bark. Saigon cinnamon.
- *kan-sui* = *gān suì* 甘遂 Euphorbia kansui root. Kan-sui.

- *ta-ky* = ***dà jǐ*** 大戟 Euphorbia pekinensis root. Peking spurge. [This traditional root, in view of its higher level of toxicity, is now usually replaced with ***hóng dà jǐ*** 紅大戟（红大戟）Knoxia valerianoides root. Knoxia.]
- *sin-chou-tsee* = ***qīng jú zi*** 青橘子（青桔子）Citrus reticulata green peel. Tangerine.

7.36g [of each].

Reduce to a powder.

- graisse de cochon = ***lard.***   *about ½ lb/250g.*
- miel = ***honey.***   *72g.*
- ***hot water.***

> § **Fr 16.1** *Nieoui-y-pou-hia.*
>
> Maladie de la vache qui a mis bas; le placenta du veau n'est pas tombé, l'animal ne mange pas, ne remue pas.

§ **Tr 16.1** *nuí yī bù xià*
牛醫不下（牛医不下）
treating a cow for [placenta] not coming down
(= retained placenta)

A disorder of a cow which has calved; the calf's placenta has not emerged, the animal does not eat & does not move.

Fr 16.2 Retirer avec la main le placenta, et donner *chin-chang-san.* – *Tchuen-chin-kia, ta-ky, hay-kin-cha, hoa-che*; réduire en poudre; graisse de porc (150ᵍ), eau chaude.

Tr 16.2 Extract the placenta by hand, and *give* :- **qīng chǎng sǎn** 清場散（清场散）*Clearing-out Powder*:

- *tchuen-chin-kia* = **chuān shān jiǎ** 穿山甲 Pangolin scales.
- *ta-ky* = **dà jǐ** 大戟 Euphorbia pekinensis root. Peking spurge. [This traditional root, in view of its higher level of toxicity, is now usually replaced with **hóng dà jǐ** 紅大戟（红大戟）Knoxia valerianoides root. Knoxia.]
- *hay-kin-cha* = **hǎi jīn shā** 海金沙 Lygodium japonicum spores. Lygodium.
- *hoa-che* = **huá shí** 滑石 Talcum.

[quantities unstated].

Reduce to a powder.

41

- graisse de porc = *lard.*   *150g.*
- *hot water.*

> ## § Fr 17.1   *Py-jou-seng-tchoang.*
>
> Boutons sur tout le corps, comme *kiai-tchoang* ; oppression, tête basse, émission de sang par les voies urinaires.

§ Tr 17.1   *pí rú shēn chuāng*
脾濡身瘡（脾濡身疮）
splenic moist generalized sores

Papules all over the body, like *scabies* (*kiai-tchoang* = **jiè chuāng** 疥瘡, 疥疮); breathlessness, head low, passage of blood in the urine.

Fr 17.2 Donner *yu-kin-san.* — *Yu-kin, kou-seng, ma-houang, jin-seng, po-ho, cha-seng, kan-tsao* ($7^g,36$); réduire en poudre; miel (150^g), eau chaude.

Tr 17.2 *Give* :- **yù jīn săn** 鬱金散（郁金散）*Turmeric Powder*:

- *yu-kin* = **yù jīn** 鬱金（郁金）Curcuma spp. root. *Inc.* turmeric.
- *kou-seng* = **kŭ shēn** 苦參（苦参）Sophora flavescens root. Flavescent sophora.
- *ma-houang* = **má huáng** 麻黃（麻黄）Ephedra spp. leaf/stem. Ephedra.
- *jin-seng* = **rén shēn** 人參（人参）Panax ginseng root. Ginseng.
- *po-ho* = **bò hé** 薄荷 Mentha haplocalyx herb. Field mint.
- *cha-seng* = **shā shēn** 沙參（沙参）1. Glehnia littoralis root. Glehnia. 2. Adenophora stricta root. Adenophora.
- *kan-tsao* = **gān căo** 甘草（甘艹）Glycyrrhiza spp. root. Licorice. Liquorice.

7.36g [of each].

Reduce to a powder.

- miel = *honey.*   *150g.*
- *hot water.*

§ **Fr 18.1**   *Sse-ky-tcheou-py.*

Agitation, oppression, somnolence, tête basse; l'animal se couche; langue pendante, eau coulant par les naseaux, boutons dans l'oreille.

§ **Tr 18.1**   *shī qì xū pí*
濕氣虛脾(湿气虚脾)
damp Qi & spleen vacuity

Restlessness, breathlessness, drowsiness, head low; the animal lies down; tongue hangs out, water flows from the nostrils, papules in the ear.

Fr 18.2 Remède : *Seng-kiang, ling-yu-san, ping-lang, to-ho, pe-tchou, kan-tsao, hiang-fou-tsee, houei-sing, fou-tsee, tsang-chou* (11ᵍ); réduire en poudre, eau chaude.

Tr 18.2 Remedy :-
- *Seng-kiang* = **shēng jiāng** 生薑(生姜) Zingibcr officinalis fresh rhizome. Ginger.
- *ling-yu-san* = **líng yú săn** 零榆散 Ulmus pumila inner bark powder. Siberian elm.
- *ping-lang* = **bīng láng** 檳榔(槟榔) Areca catechu nut. Betel.
- *to-ho* = **tù hé** 菟核 Amelopsis japonica fruit/root. Japanese peppervine.
- *pe-tchou* = **bái chŏu** 白丑 Pharbitis spp. seed. Morning glory.
- *kan-tsao* = **gān căo** 甘草(甘艸) Glycyrrhiza spp. root. Licorice. Liquorice.

45

- *hiang-fou-tsee* = **xiāng fù zǐ** 香附子 Cyperus rotundus rhizome. Nut-grass.
- *houei-sing* = **huī xiàn** 灰莧(灰苋) Chenopodium album seed. Pigweed.
- *fou-tsee* = **fù zǐ** 附子 Aconitum carmichaeli prepared accessory root. Sichuan aconite.
- *tsang-chou* = **cháng chǔ** 萇楚苌楚 Actinidia chinensis/rufa fruit. A type of kiwi fruit.

11g [of each].

Reduce to a powder.

- **hot water.**

> **§ Fr 19.1** *Hin-tsao-pou-tchuen.*
>
> Selles mélangées de sang, ventre enflé, l'animal frappe la terre avec les pieds, souffle bruyant par les naseaux; plaintes, inappétence.

§ Tr 19.1 *xīng cǎo bù chuān*
驿艸不穿（驿草不穿）
brownish red straw, without a penetrating wound

Stools mixed with blood, belly swollen, the animal stamps on the ground, noisy breathing through the nostrils; groaning, lack of appetite.

Fr 19.2 Traitement : *Sin-ky-san.* — *Ping-lang, hoa-che, tsien-lieou, ta-ky, hoang-tsin, hoang-ky, ta-hoang, po-siao* (11ᵍ); réduire en poudre; graisse de porc (200ᵍ); eau chaude.

Tr 19.2 Treatment :- **xīn qì sǎn** 心氣散（心气散） *Heart Qi Powder*:

- *ping-lang* = **bīng láng** 檳榔（槟榔） Areca catechu nut. Betel.
- *hoa-che* = **huá shí** 滑石 Talcum.
- *tsien-lieou* = **chēng liǔ** 檉柳（柽柳） Tamarix chinensis twig & leaf. Tamarisk.
- *ta-ky* = **dà jǐ** 大戟 Euphorbia pekinensis root. Peking spurge. [This traditional root, in view of its higher level of toxicity, is now usually replaced with **hóng dà jǐ** 紅大戟（红大戟） Knoxia valerianoides root. Knoxia.]
- *hoang-tsin* = **huáng qín** 黃芩（黄芩） Scutellaria baicalensis root. Baical skullcap.
- *hoang-ky* = **huáng qí** 黃芪（黄芪） Astragalus spp. root. Milk vetch.

- *ta-hoang* = ***dà huáng*** 大黃（大黃）Rheum spp. root/rhizome. Rhubarb.
- *po-siao* = ***pǔ xiāo*** 朴消 Glauber's salt. Mirabilite.

11g [of each].

Reduce to a powder.

- graisse de porc = ***lard.***   *200g.*
- ***hot water.***

§ **Fr 20.1**   *Jou-fen-toui-nio.*

Oppression, yeux rouges, langue sèche, inappétence, somno-lence, pouls tombant.

§ **Tr 20.1**   *rú fèn tuī niào*
濡糞推尿（濡粪推尿）
wet stools & delayed urination

Breathlessness, red eyes, dry tongue, lack of appetite, drowsiness, fading-away [weak] pulse.

Fr 20.2 *Ou-kia-san.* — *Ma-hoang, ou-teou, kan-choui-che, che-kao, yuen-kin-che* (72^g); pulvériser; graisse de porc (400^g), eau chaude; et si ce reméde ne réussit pas, après deux fois, ajouter *ta-hoang* (2^g).

Tr 20.2 Treatment :- ***wú xiè sǎn*** 無瀉散（无泻散）*No Diarrhoea Powder*:

- *ma-hoang* = ***má huáng*** 麻黄（麻黄）Ephedra spp. leaf/stem. Ephedra.
- *ou-teou* = ***wū tóu*** 烏頭（乌头）Aconitum carmichaeli prepared accessory root. Sichuan aconite.
- *kan-choui-che* = ***kǎn shuǐ shí*** 坎水石 Selenite. Crystalline gypsum (gypsum flower).
- *che-kao* = ***shí gāo*** 石膏 Crystalline gypsum.
- *yuen-kin-che* = ***yuán qín qiē*** 元芩切 Scutellaria baicalensis root slices. Baical skullcap.

72g [of each].

Reduce to a powd

- graisse de porc = **lard.**   *400g.*
- **hot water.**

Should this remedy be unsuccessful after two doses, add:

- *ta-hoang* = **dà huáng*** 大黃（大黃）Rheum spp. root/rhizome. Rhubarb.

                                                                                                    2g.

[*According to Bensky et al, whereas large doses (≥ *10g*) are purgative, small doses (< *10g*) have the opposite effect.]

§ **Fr 21.1** *Lieou-kouai-jĕ-ping.*

Le bœuf se couche et dort; inappétence, oppression, langue bleue; il ne veut pas bouger.

§ **Tr 21.1** *liú kuài rè bìng*
流快熱病（流快热病）
rapid flow heat disease

The ox gets down & lies still; lack of appetite, breathlessness, blue tongue; he does not want to budge.

Fr 21.2 Remède : *San-hiang-san. — Hoang-yo-tsee, tche-mou-pe, yo-tsee, pe-mou, ta-hoang, hoang-tsin, kan-tsao, yu-kin* (7ᵍ,36); pulvériser; eau chaude.

Tr 21.2 Remedy :- ***sàn xiāng săn*** 散香散 *Fragrant Dissipating Powder*:

- *hoang-yo-tsee* = ***huáng yào zǐ*** 黃藥子（黄药子） Discorea bulbifera rhizome (tuber). Air yam/potato.

- *tche-mou-pe* = ***zhī mǔ bèi*** 知母備（知母备） Anemarrhena asphodeloides prepared rhizome. Anemarrhena.

- *yo-tsee* = ***yǔ sī*** 雨絲（雨丝） Tamarix chinensis stem & leaves. Tamarisk.

- *pe-mou* = ***bèi mǔ*** 貝母（贝母） Fritillaria spp. bulb. Fritillary.

- *ta-hoang* = ***dà huáng*** 大黃（大黄） Rheum spp. root/rhizome. Rhubarb.

- *hoang-tsin* = ***huáng qín*** 黃芩（黄芩） Scutellaria baicalensis root. Baical skullcap.

- *kan-tsao* = ***gān căo*** 甘草（甘艸） Glycyrrhiza spp. root. Licorice. Liquorice.

- *yu-kin* = **yù jīn** 鬱金（郁金）Curcuma spp. root. *Inc.* turmeric.

  7.36g [of each].

  Reduce to a powder.

- **hot water.**

> **§ Fr 22.1** *Cha-che-ling.*
>
> Queue en l'air, tête basse, l'animal se couche, urine mêlée de gravier; lassitude, inappétence, plaintes.

§ Tr 22.1

qiǎ shí lín
卡石淋
obstructing stone strangury

Tail in the air, head low, the animal lies down, urine mixed with gravel; lassitude, lack of appetite, groaning.

Fr 22.2 Saignier, donner ensuite *tsin-tche-san.* – *Hoa-che, mou-tong, yen-choui-tsee, houei-sin, ho-po, to-ho, pe-tchou, hoang-tsin, he-tsien-lieou* (7ᵍ,36); pulvériser; eau chaude.

Tr 22.2 *Bleed, then give* :- **qīng zhì sǎn** 清滯散（清滞散）*Clearing Stagnation Powder*:

- *hoa-che* = **huá shí** 滑石 Talcum.
- *mou-tong* = **mù tōng** 木通 Akebia spp. stalk. Akebia.
- *yen-choui-tsee* = **yún shuǐ shí** 雲水石（云水石）Carbonate of lime.
- *houei-sin* = **huī xiàn** 灰莧（灰苋）Chenopodium album seed. Pigweed.
- *ho-po* = **hòu pò** 厚朴 Magnolia officinalis bark. Magnolia.
- *to-ho* = **tù hé** 菟核 Amelopsis japonica fruit/root. Japanese peppervine.
- *pe-tchou* = **bái chǒu** 白丑 Pharbitis spp. seed. Morning glory.
- *hoang-tsin* = **huáng qín** 黃芩（黄芩）Scutellaria baicalensis root. Baical skullcap.

- *he-tsien-lieou* = **hé chēng liǔ** 河檉柳（河柽柳） Tamarix chinensis twig & leaf. Tamarisk.

7.36g [of each].

Reduce to a powder.

- **hot water.**

§ **Fr 23.1**   *Nieou-kouan, kien-ty-ping.*

    Blessure à la jambe, enflure.

§ **Tr 23.1**   *niú guǎn : jiān dī bìng*
牛管 湔滌病（牛管 湔涤病）
cattle husbandry : washing imperfections

Leg wounds, swelling.

Fr 23.2 Donner *jou-hiang-san*. — *Jou-hiang, long-kou, hoang-tan, che-hiang,* cheveux torréfiés, *tchou-cha* (7ᵍ,36); pulvériser; eau, lotions d'eau fraiche.

Tr 23.2 *Give* :- **rù xiāng sǎn** 乳香散 *Frankincense Powder*:
- *jou-hiang* = **rù xiāng** 乳香 Olibanum. Frankincense.
- *long-kou* = **lóng gǔ** 龍骨（龙骨）Dragon bone. Fossil bone.
- *hoang-tan* = **huáng dān** 黃丹（黄丹）Massicot. Yellow lead oxide.
- *che-hiang* = **shè xiāng** 麝香 Moschus. Musk.
- cheveux torréfiés = Torrefied hair,
- *tchou-cha* = **zhū shā** 朱砂 Cinnabar. Red mercury sulphide.

7.36g [of each].

Reduce to a powder.

- **water.**

[Apply as] fresh water lotions.

§ **Fr 24.1**   *Po-chang-fong.*

Lassitude, sang coulant par les naseaux et par la bouche; l'animal se couche.

§ **Tr 24.1**   *bó cháng fēng*
搏腸風（搏肠风）
contends with intestine wind

Lassitude, blood flowing from the nostrils and mouth; the animal lies down.

Fr 24.2 Remède : ~~Tien-ma-san, tien-ma,~~ *Tien-ma-san. – Tien-ma, ty-yu, tchuen-hiong, tche-mou, ou-che, pan-hia, tchou-cha* (4^g); *vin et eau.*

Tr 24.2 Remedy :- **tiān má săn** 天麻散 *Gastrodia Powder*:

- *tien-ma* = **tiān má** 天麻 Gastrodia elata rhizome. Gastrodia.
- *ty-yu* = **dì yú** 地榆 Sanguisorba officinalis root. Burnet-bloodwort.
- *tchuen-hiong* = **chuān xiōng** 川芎 Ligusticum chuanxiong rhizome. Sichuan lovage root.
- *tche-mou* = **zhī mŭ** 知母 Anemarrhena asphodeloides rhizome. Anemarrhena.
- *ou-che* = **wū shé** 烏蛇（乌蛇）Zaocys dhumnades. Blackstriped snake.
- *pan-hia* = **bàn xià** 半夏 Pinellia ternata rhizome. Pinellia.
- *tchou-cha* = **zhū shā** 朱砂 Cinnabar. Red mercury sulphide.

4g [of each].

- **wine & water.**

§ Fr 25.1   *Su-fong-ty-ping.*

Delire; l'animal court comme un furieux, plaintes; il mord la terre; de l'eau jaune coule par la bouche; movements des mâchoires.

§ Tr 25.1   *sōu fēng dì bìng*
                    搜風地病(搜风地病)
                    track down wind earth disease

Delirium; the animal runs about as though enraged, groaning; it bites the earth; yellow water flows from the mouth; movements of the jaw.

Fr 25.2 Traitement : *Tchin-sin-san. — Fou-ling, yuen-tche, hong-tsin, tche-mou, pe-mou, tsee-tsee, ho-py, jou-hiang, po-siao* (7ᵍ,36), *miel* (72ᵍ); *eau chaude.*

Tr 25.2   Treatment :- **quīng xīn sǎn** 清心散 *Clearing Heart Powder*:

- *fou-ling* = **fú líng** 茯苓 Poria cocos. Poria. China root.
- *yuen-tche* = **yuǎn zhì** 遠志(远志) Polygala spp. root. Thinleaf milkwort.
- *hong-tsin* = **hóng shēn** 紅參(红参) Panax ginseng root. Red ginseng.
- *tche-mou* = **zhī mǔ** 知母 Anemarrhena asphodeloides rhizome. Anemarrhena.
- *pe-mou* = **bèi mǔ** 貝母(贝母) Fritillaria spp. bulb. Fritillary.
- *tsee-tsee* = **zhī zǐ** 栀子(栀子) Gardenia jasminoides fruit. Cape jasmine.
- *ho-py* = **hé bí** 荷鼻 Nelumbo nucifera leaf stalk. Lotus.
- *jou-hiang* = **rù xiāng** 乳香 Olibanum. Frankincense.

- *po-siao* = ***pǔ xiāo*** 朴消 Glauber's salt. Mirabilite.

  7.36g [of each].

  Reduce to a powder.

- miel = ***honey.***   *72g.*
- ***hot water.***

> **§ Fr 26.1**   *Je-fey-ping.*
>
> Oppression; l'animal se couche sur le dos les quatre pieds en l'air; mouvements des mâchoires, mucosités coulant par la bouche et les naseaux

§ Tr 26.1

rè fèi bìng

熱肺病（热肺病）

hot lung disease

Breathlessness; the animal lies on its back with all four feet in the air; movements of the jaw, mucus flowing from the mouth and nostrils.

Fr 26.2 Remède : *Che-hiang-san.* — Musc (0ᵍ,03), *hoang-tan* (20ᵍ), *mo-yo* (11ᵍ), *ou-kong* (20ᵍ), *pi-choang* (0ᵍ,03), *kou-fan* (0ᵍ,04); pulvériser, eau.

Tr 26.2   Remedy :- ***shí xiāng sǎn*** 石香散 *Fragrant Mineral Powder*:

- Musc = ***shè xiāng*** 麝香 Moschus. Musk.   *0.03g [30mg].*

- *hoang-tan* = ***huáng dān*** 黃丹（黄丹）Massicot. Yellow lead oxide.   *20g.*

- *mo-yo* = ***mò yào*** 沒藥（沒药）Myrrh.   *11g.*

- *ou-kong* = ***wú gōng*** 蜈蚣 Scolopendra. Centipede.   *20g.*

- *pi-choang* = ***pī shuāng*** 砒霜 Sublimed arsenic.   *0.03g [30mg].*

- *kou-fan* = ***kū fán*** 枯礬 (枯矾) Calcined alum.

  0.04g [40mg].

  Reduce to a powder.

- ***water.***

> ## § Fr 27.1 *Nieou-hoang-py-piang.*
>
> L'animal frappe la terre avec les pieds; diarrhée, en même temps émission d'urine pendant la selle; langue ~~noirâtre~~ noirâtre.

§ Tr 27.1

niú huáng pí biàn
牛黃脾便（牛黄脾便）
cow's yellow spleen stool

The animal stamps on the ground; diarrhoea; at the same time, micturition during defaecation; tongue blackish.

Fr 27.2 *Pe-kouei-san. — Pe-tchou, tsang-chou, tsee-yuen, tang-kouei, ma-hoang, ho-po, nieou-sy, ho-pen* (7^g,36); eau chaude

Tr 27.2 *[Give]* :- **bái guì săn** 白貴散（白贵散）*Precious White Powder*:

- *pe-tchou* = **bái chŏu** 白丑 Pharbitis spp. seed. Morning glory.
- *tsang-chou* = **cháng chŭ** 萇楚（苌楚）Actinidia chinensis/rufa fruit. A type of kiwi fruit.
- *tsee-yuen* = **zǐ yuàn** 紫菀 Aster tartaricus root. Purple aster.
- *tang-kouei* = **dāng guī** 當歸（当归）Angelica sinensis root. Chinese angelica.
- *ma-hoang* = **má huáng** 麻黃（麻黄）Ephedra spp. leaf/stem. Ephedra.
- *ho-po* = **hòu pò** 厚朴 Magnolia officinalis bark. Magnolia.
- *nieou-sy* = **niú xī** 牛膝 Achyranthes bidentata root. Achyranthes.

- *ho-pen* = **hóu bǎn [lì]** 猴板〔栗〕 Aesculus spp. nut. Horse chestnut.

  7.36g [of each].

  Reduce to a powder.

- **hot water.**

§ **Fr 28.1** *Fey-tong-pa-py.*

L'animal se couche; amaigrissement, lassitude, inappétence, mouvements des mâchoires, botborygmes.

§ **Tr 28.1** *fèi tōng bǎ pí*
肺通把脾
freeing lung takes hold of spleen

The animal lies down; emaciation, lassitude, lack of appetite, movements of the jaw, rumbling bowels.

Fr 28.2 Remède : *Pan-hia-san.* — *Pan-hia, tche-mou, pe-mou, tsang-chou, pe-tsee, sy-sin, kou-fen, tchuen-hiong, hoang-tsin* (7^g,36); poudre; ajouter vin, gingembre, eau chaude.

Tr 28.2 Remedy :- ***bàn xià sǎn*** 半夏散 *Pinellia Powder*:
- *pan-hia* = ***bàn xià*** 半夏 Pinellia ternata rhizome. Pinellia.
- *tche-mou* = ***zhī mǔ*** 知母 Anemarrhena asphodeloides rhizome. Anemarrhena.
- *pe-mou* = ***bèi mǔ*** 貝母（贝母）Fritillaria spp. bulb. Fritillary.
- *tsang-chou* = ***cháng chǔ*** 萇楚（苌楚）Actinidia chinensis/rufa fruit. A type of kiwi fruit.
- *pe-tsee* = ***bái zhǐ*** 白芷 Angelica dahurica root. Dahurican angelica.
- *sy-sin* = ***xì xīn*** 細辛（细辛）Asarum spp. root/rhizome. Chinese wild ginger.
- *kou-fen* = ***kū fán*** 枯礬（枯矾）Calcined alum.
- *tchuen-hiong* = ***chuān xiōng*** 川芎 Ligusticum chuanxiong rhizome. Sichuan lovage root.

63

- *hoang-tsin* = ***huáng qín*** 黄芩 (黃芩) Scutellaria baicalensis root. Baical skullcap.

7.36g [of each].

[Reduce to] powder.

Add :-
- ***wine.***
- gingembre = ***ginger.***
- ***hot water.***

§ **Fr 29.1**   *Tsuen-y-ping.*

Poils hérissés, ventre enflé, délire furieux.

§ **Tr 29.1**   *chuān yì bìng*
                                           川疫病
                                    Sichuan epidemic disease

Hair stands on end, swollen belly, raging frenzy.

Fr 29.2 Remède : *Jin-seng-san. — Cho-yo, jin-seng, hoang-tsin, pe-mou, tche-mou, yu-kin, fang-fong, pe-fan, hoang-lien, kiĕ-keng, hoa-lo, ta-hoang, tsee-tsee* (7ᵍ,36); réduire en poudre; sucre (150ᵍ), gingembre (400ᵍ); pulvériser; eau chaude.

Tr 29.2   Remedy :- **rén shēn săn** 人參散（人参散）*Ginseng Powder*:

- *cho-yo* = **sháo yào** 芍藥（芍药）Paeonia spp. rubra root. Red peony root.
- *jin-seng* = **rén shēn** 人參（人参）Panax ginseng root. Ginseng.
- *hoang-tsin* = **huáng qín** 黃芩（黄芩）Scutellaria baicalensis root. Baical skullcap.
- *pe-mou* = **bèi mŭ** 貝母（贝母）Fritillaria spp. bulb. Fritillary.
- *tche-mou* = **zhī mŭ** 知母 Anemarrhena asphodeloides rhizome. Anemarrhena.
- *yu-kin* = **yù jīn** 鬱金（郁金）Curcuma spp. root. *Inc.* turmeric.
- *fang-fong* = **fáng fēng** 防風（防风）Saposhnikovia divaricata root. Saposhnikovia.
- *pe-fan* = **bái fán** 白礬（白矾）Alum.

- *hoang-lien* = **huáng lián** 黄連(黄连) Coptis spp. rhizome. Goldthread.
- *kiě-keng* = **jié gěng** 桔梗 Platycodon grandiflorus root. Balloon flower.
- *hoa-lo* = **guā lóu** 瓜蔞(瓜蒌) Trichosanthes kirilowii/ rosthornii fruit. Chinese cucumber.
- *ta-hoang* = **dà huáng** 大黄(大黄) Rheum spp. root/rhizome. Rhubarb.
- *tsee-tsee* = **zhī zǐ** 栀子(栀子) Gardenia jasminoides fruit. Cape jasmine.

7.36g [of each].

Reduce to a powder.

[*Add* :-]

- sucre = **sugar.**   *150g.*
- gingembre = **ginger.**   *400g.*

[Reduce to] powder.

- **hot water.**

§ Fr 30.1   *Kiao-fong-ping.*

L'animal ne peut plus remuer les pieds, inappétence, il tourne continuellement la tête; mouvements des mâchoires, écoulement d'eau jaune par la bouche.

§ Tr 30.1   *jiāo fēng bìng*
                          焦風病(焦风病)
                          burner wind disease

The animal can no longer move its feet, lack of appetite, it continually turns its head; movements of the jaw, a flow of yellow water from the mouth.

Fr 30.2 Remède : *Tchou-fong-san. — Ou-che, kan-siě, tsai-tou, ho-po, tang-kouei, ma-hoang, tchuen-hiong, ou-to, houei-sin, fang-fong, pe-fou-tsee, tien-tong* (7ᵍ,36); pulvériser; eau chaude, un peu de vin.
*

Tr 30.2 Treatment :- ***chú fēng sǎn*** 除風散(除风散) *Eliminate Wind Powder*:

- *ou-che* = ***wū shé*** 烏蛇(乌蛇) Zaocys dhumnades. Blackstriped snake.
- *kan-siě* = ***gān zhè*** 甘蔗 Sugar cane.
- *tsai-tou* = ***cài dòu*** 菜豆 Phaseolus vulgaris seed. Kidney bean.
- *ho-po* = ***hòu pò*** 厚朴 Magnolia officinalis bark. Magnolia.
- *tang-kouei* = ***dāng guī*** 當歸(当归) Angelica sinensis root. Chinese angelica.
- *ma-hoang* = ***má huáng*** 麻黃(麻黄) Ephedra spp. leaf/stem. Ephedra.

67

- *tchuen-hiong* = **chuān xiōng** 川芎 Ligusticum chuanxiong rhizome. Sichuan lovage root.
- *ou-to* = **wū tóu** 烏頭（乌头）Aconitum carmichaeli prepared accessory root. Sichuan aconite.
- *houei-sin* = **huī xiàn** 灰莧（灰苋）Chenopodium album seed. Pigweed.
- *fang-fong* = **fáng fēng** 防風（防风）Saposhnikovia divaricata root. Saposhnikovia.
- *pe-fou-tsee* = **bái fù zǐ** 白附子 Typhonium giganteum prepared rhizome. Giant voodoo lily.
- *tien-tong* = **tiān dōng** 天冬 Asparagus cochinchinensis tuber. Asparagus.

7.36g [of each].

Reduce to a powder.

- **hot water.**
- **a little wine.**

> **§ Fr 31.1**   *Fey-pe-ty-ping.*
>
> Jambes courbées, l'animal ne marche pas; oppression; des mucosités purulentes coulentb par les naseaux.

§ Tr 31.1   *fèi bái tì bìng*
肺白涕病
lung white nasal mucus disease

Legs bent, the animal does not walk; breathlessness; purulent mucus flows from the nostrils.

Fr 31.2 Remède : *Hing-jin-san. — Hing-jin, po-ho, hoa-lo, tche-mou, pe-mou, sin-kiao, tsee-tsee, kiang-kiun* (7ᵍ,36); réduire en poudre; miel (100ᵍ); eau chaude.

Tr 31.2 Remedy :- Treatment :- **xìng rén sǎn** 杏仁散 *Apricot Kernel Powder* (formula differs from that given in **1.2** above):

- *hing-jin* = **xìng rén** 杏仁 Prunus spp. seed/kernel. Apricot.
- *po-ho* = **bò hé** 薄荷 Mentha haplocalyx herb. Field mint.
- *hoa-lo* = **guā lóu** 瓜蔞(瓜蒌) Trichosanthes kirilowii/ rosthornii fruit. Chinese cucumber.
- *tche-mou* = **zhī mǔ** 知母 Anemarrhena asphodeloides rhizome. Anemarrhena.
- *pe-mou* = **bèi mǔ** 貝母(贝母) Fritillaria spp. bulb. Fritillary.
- *sin-kiao* = **qín jiāo** 秦艽 Gentiana spp. root. Large gentian.
- *tsee-tsee* = **zhī zǐ** 梔子(栀子) Gardenia jasminoides fruit. Cape jasmine.

- *kiang-kiun* = ***jiāng jūn*** 將軍（将军）Rheum spp.
  root/rhizome. Rhubarb.

  7.36g [of each].

  Reduce to a powder.

- miel = ***honey.*** *100g.*
- ***hot water.***

§ **Fr 32.1**   *Nieou-che-ping.*

Langue enflée et dure, bouche ulcerée, borborygmes.

§ **Tr 32.1**   *niú shí bìng*
牛時病（牛时病）
cow's seasonal disease

Swollen & hard tongue, ulcerated mouth, rumbling bowels.

Fr 32.2 Remède : *Ya-siao-san. — Ya-siao, kan-tsao, hoang-tsin, yu-kin, ta-hoang, houang-lien, po-siao* (7ᵍ,36), miel (150ᵍ), graisse de porc (150ᵍ), eau chaude.

Tr 32.2 Treatment :- ***yá xiāo săn*** 牙消散 *Nitre Powder*:

- *ya-siao* = ***yá xiāo*** 牙消 Horse-tooth nitre/niter. Saltpetre/Saltpeter.
- *kan-tsao* = ***gān căo*** 甘草（甘艸）Glycyrrhiza spp. root. Licorice. Liquorice.
- *hoang-tsin* = ***huáng qín*** 黄芩（黄芩）Scutellaria baicalensis root. Baical skullcap.
- *yu-kin* = ***yù jīn*** 鬱金（郁金）Curcuma spp. root. *Inc.* turmeric.
- *ta-hoang* = ***dà huáng*** 大黄（大黄）Rheum spp. root/rhizome. Rhubarb.
- *houang-lien* = ***huáng lián*** 黄連（黄连）Coptis spp. rhizome. Goldthread.
- *po-siao* = ***pǔ xiāo*** 朴消 Glauber's salt. Mirabilite.

7.36g [of each].

71

- miel = ***honey.***   *150g.*
- grasse de porc = ***lard.***   *150g.*
- ***hot water.***

§ **Fr 33.1**   *Choang-pou-ping.*

Jambes enflées, l'animal ne peut marcher, inappétence, somnolence.

§ **Tr 33.1**   *zhàng bǒ bìng*
脹跛病（胀跛病）
dropsical lameness disease

Swollen legs, the animal is unable to walk, lack of appetite, drowsiness.

Fr 33.2 Remède : *Kin-kien-tsao-san. — My-to-seng, fou-tsee, ou-che, tsao-hoa, tang-kouei, pie-kia* (7^g,36); pulvériser; eau chaude avec un peu de vin.

Tr 33.2   Treatment :- ***jīn jiàn cǎo sǎn*** 金鑒艸散（金鉴草散） *Golden Mirror Herb Powder*:

- *my-to-seng* = ***mì tuó sēng*** 密陀僧 Litharge. Impure lead oxide.
- *fou-tsee* = ***fù zǐ*** 附子 Aconitum carmichaeli prepared accessory root. Sichuan aconite.
- *ou-che* = ***wū shé*** 烏蛇（乌蛇）Zaocys dhumnades. Blackstriped snake.
- *tsao-hoa* = ***cǎo hāo*** 艸蒿（草蒿）Artemisia annua leaves, stem, & whole herb. Sweet womwood.
- *tang-kouei* = ***dāng guī*** 當歸（当归）Angelica sinensis root. Chinese angelica.
- *pie-kia* = ***bì xiè*** 萆薢（萆薢）Dioscorea collettii rhizome. Fish-poison yam.

7.36g [of each].

Reduce to a powder.

- *hot water.*
- *a little wine.*

§ **Fr 34.1** *Lao-ping.*

Maigreur extrême, le bœuf ne veut pas travailler, chaleur, inappétence, plaintes, mouvements des mâchoires; quelquefois il s'agenouille; ventre enflé.

§ **Tr 34.1** *láo bìng*
勞病（劳病）
taxation disease

Extreme thinness, the ox does not want to work, hot, lack of appetite, groaning, movements of the jaws; sometimes he kneels down; swollen belly.

Fr 34.2 Remède : *Ta-ky-san. — Hiu-choui-tsee, ho-po, mou-tong, kien-lieou, hoa-che, kouei-hiang, tchuen-lien-tsee, pe-tchou, houei-sin, hay-kin-cha* (4^g) ou *hiang-yeou* (7^g,36); pulvériser; eau chaude.

Tr 34.2 Treatment :- **dà qì sǎn** 大氣散（大气散）*Major Qi Powder*:

- *hiu-choui-tsee* = **xù suí zǐ** 續隨子（续随子）Euphorbia lathyris seed/herb/flower. Caper spurge.
- *ho-po* = **hòu pò** 厚朴 Magnolia officinalis bark. Magnolia.
- *mou-tong* = **mù tōng** 木通 Akebia spp. stalk. Akebia.
- *kien-lieou* = **jiàn [yè] liǔ** 箭［葉］蓼（箭［叶］蓼）Polygonum sieboldii seed/entire. Smartweed.
- *hoa-che* = **huá shí** 滑石 Talcum.
- *kouei-hiang* = **guǐ jiàn** 鬼箭 Euonymus alatus 'wings'/twigs. Spindle tree.
- *tchuen-lien-tsee* = **chuān liàn zǐ** 川楝子 Melia toosendan fruit. Sichuan pagoda tree.

- *pe-tchou* = **bái chǒu** 白丑 Pharbitis spp. seed. Morning glory.
- *houei-sin* = **huī xiàn** 灰苋(灰苋) Chenopodium album seed. Pigweed.
- *hay-kin-cha* = **hǎi jīn shā** 海金沙 Lygodium japonicum spores. Lygodium.

4g [of each].

Reduce to a powder.

Instead of Lygodium add [to the powder] :-

- *hiang-yeou* = **xiāng yóu** 香油 Sesame oil.　　　　*7.36g.*

- **hot water.**

§ **Fr 35.1**   *Ouei-fan-ty-ping.*

Vomissements de matières bilieuses, plaintes; l'animal ne remue pas et s'agenouille.

§ **Tr 35.1**   *wèi fǎn dí bìng*
胃反滌病（胃反涤病）
stomach reflex flushing disease

Vomiting of bilious matter, groaning; the animal does not move and kneels.

Fr 35.2 Saigner; donner *pou-hoang-san.* — *Kouai-kouei, ho-po, kouei-hiang, tsin-py, kan-tsao, tchin-py, tsang-chou, ou-oey-tsee, pe-tchou, mou-hiang, mou-kouei* (7ᵍ,36); pulvériser.

Tr 35.2 *Bleed; then give* :- **bù huang sǎn** 不黃散（不黄散）*No Jaundice Powder*:

- *kouai-kouei* = **gài guī** 蓋龜（盖龟）Turtle shell.
- *ho-po* = **hòu pò** 厚朴 Magnolia officinalis bark. Magnolia.
- *kouei-hiang* = **guǐ jiàn** 鬼箭 Euonymus alatus 'wings'/twigs. Spindle tree.
- *tsin-py* = **qīng pí** 青皮 Citrus reticulata green peel. Tangerine.
- *kan-tsao* = = **gān cǎo** 甘草（甘艸）Glycyrrhiza spp. root. Licorice. Liquorice.
- *tchin-py* = **chén pí** 陳皮（陈皮）Citrus reticulata aged peel. Tangerine.
- *tsang-chou* = **cháng chǔ** 萇楚（苌楚）Actinidia chinensis/rufa fruit. A type of kiwi fruit.

- *ou-oey-tsee* = **wǔ wèi zǐ** 五味子 Schisandra spp. fruit. Five-flavour berry.
- *pe-tchou* = **bái chǒu** 白丑 Pharbitis spp. seed. Morning glory.
- *mou-hiang* = **mù xiāng** 木香 Aucklandia lappa root. Saussurea.
- *mou-kouei* = **mù gui** 木桂 Cinnamomum cassia unscraped bark of larger tree. Cinnamon.

7.36g [of each].

Reduce to a powder.

> **§ Fr 36.1**   *Fey-lao-ping.*
>
> Le bœuf a les yeux fermés, il ne peut lever les pieds, mouvements des mâchoires; écoulement par la bouche et par les naseaux d'une eau jaune.

§ Tr 36.1   *fèi láo bìng*
肺勞病（肺劳病）
lung taxation disease

The ox has his eyes closed, he cannot lift his feet, movements of the jaws; a discharge of yellow water from the mouth and nostrils.

Fr 36.2 Remède : *Pe-hoai-san. — Kan-tsao, ou-yo, pe-mou, ma-teou-ling, hoang-tsin, pe-fan, tche-mou, san-pe-py* (7ᵍ,36); pulvériser; eau chaude, sel (7ᵍ,36).

Tr 36.2   Remedy :- ***bài huài săn*** 敗壞散（败坏散）*Vanquishing Powder*:

- *kan-tsao* = ***gān căo*** 甘草（甘艸）Glycyrrhiza spp. root. Licorice. Liquorice.
- *ou-yo* = ***wū yào*** 烏藥（乌药）Lindera aggregata root. Lindera.
- *pe-mou* = ***bèi mŭ*** 貝母（贝母）Fritillaria spp. bulb. Fritillary.
- *ma-teou-ling* = ***mă dōu líng*** 馬兜鈴（马兜铃）Aristolochia spp. fruit. Birthwort.
- *hoang-tsin* = ***huáng qín*** 黃芩（黄芩）Scutellaria baicalensis root. Baical skullcap.
- *pe-fan* = ***bái fán*** 白礬（白矾）Alum.
- *tche-mou* = ***zhī mŭ*** 知母 Anemarrhena asphodeloides rhizome. Anemarrhena.

- *san-pe-py* = ***sāng bái pí*** 桑白皮 Morus alba root bark & bark. Mulberry.

  7.36g [of each].

  Reduce to a powder.

- ***hot water.***
- sel = ***salt.***   *7.36g.*

> **§ Fr 37.1**   *Chin-chang-ping.*
>
> Douleur aux os des fesses; l'animal frappe la terre avec le pied; lassitude.oreilles basses, reins enflés, inappétence, plaintes.

§ Tr 37.1   *shèn cháng bìng*
腎腸病（肾肠病）
kidney & intestine disease

Pain in the bones of the buttocks; the animal stamps on the ground with its foot, lassitude, ears low, loins swollen, lack of appetite, groaning.

Fr 37.2 Remède : *Pou-chin-san. — Pe-tsee, tchin-py, ho-po, mo-yo, py-sie, houei-hiang, tong-kuei, tsee-jen-tong, ou-ling-tsee, lien-tsee* (7^g,36); pulvériser; gingembre (11^g); vin, eau chaude.

Tr 37.2 Remedy :- ***bǔ shèn sǎn*** 補腎散（补肾散） *Kidney-Supplementing Powder*:

- *pe-tsee* = ***bái zhǐ*** 白芷 Angelica dahurica root. Dahurican angelica.
- *tchin-py* = ***chén pí*** 陳皮（陈皮） Citrus reticulata aged peel. Tangerine.
- *ho-po* = ***hòu pò*** 厚朴 Magnolia officinalis bark. Magnolia.
- *mo-yo* = ***mò yào*** 沒藥（沒药） Myrrh.
- *py-sie* = ***pì xiè*** 萆薢 Smilax glabra root. Smilax.
- *houei-hiang* = ***huí xiāng*** 茴香 Foeniculum vulgare fruit. Fennel.
- *tong-kuei* = ***dōng kuí*** 葲葵 Malva crispa fruit. mallow.
- *tsee-jen-tong* = ***zì rán tóng*** 自然銅（自然铜） Pyrite.

- *ou-ling-tsee* = ***wǔ líng zhī*** 五靈脂（五灵脂）Flying squirrel faeces.
- *lien-tsee* = ***lián zǐ*** 蓮子（莲子）Nelumbo nucifera seed. Lotus.

7.36g [of each].

Reduce to a powder.

- gingembre = ***ginger.***　　　　　　　　　　　　　　*11g.*

- ***wine.***
- ***hot water.***

> **§ Fr 38.1** *Pao-hu-ping.*
>
> Des mucosités blanches coulent par la bouche; urine coulant goutte à goutte; maigreur, l'animal s'agenouille, oppression, plaintes.

§ Tr 38.1 *pāo xū bìng*
脬虛病（脬虚病）
bladder vacuity disease

White mucus flows from the mouth; urine dripping; thinness, the animal kneels, breathlessness, groaning.

Fr 38.2 Saignier; donner *cho-yo-san.* — *Cho-yo. tchou-yu, tang-kouei, sy-sin, jou-kouei, long-kou,* sel (7ᵍ,36), pulvériser; huile (36ᵍ) eau chaude.

Tr 38.2 Remedy :- ***sháo yào sǎn*** 芍藥散（芍药散）*Peony Powder*:

- *cho-yo* = ***sháo yào*** 芍藥（芍药）Paeonia spp. rubra root. Red peony root.
- *tchou-yu* = ***zhú yóu*** 竹油 Bamboo spp. sap (dried).
- *tang-kouei* = ***dāng guī*** 當歸（当归）Angelica sinensis root. Chinese angelica.
- *sy-sin* = ***xì xīn*** 細辛（细辛）Asarum spp. root/rhizome. Chinese wild ginger.
- *jou-kouei* = ***ròu guì*** 肉桂 Cinnamomum cassia inner bark. Saigon cinnamon.
- *long-kou* = ***lóng gǔ*** 龍骨（龙骨）Dragon bone. Fossil bone.
- sel = ***salt.***

7.36g [of each].

Reduce to a powder.

- huile = *oil.*   *36g.*
- *hot water.*

§ **Fr 39.1**   *Han-choang-hoang.*

Souffle bruyant par les naseaux, râle dans la gorge, chaleur, cou enflé, mouvements des mâchoires, écoulement de mucosités purulentes et mêlée de sang par la bouche; l'animal se couche, inappétence.

§ **Tr 39.1**   *gān zhàng huáng*
肝脹黃（肝胀黄）
liver yellow swelling

Noisy breathing through the nostrils, rattling in the throat, heat, swelling in the neck, jaw movements, discharge of purulent mucus mixed with blood from the mouth; the animal lies down, lack of appetite.

Fr 39.2 Saigner. *Nan-pong-cha-san. — Nan-pong-cha, hoang-lien, jin-seng, po-ho, tchuen-hiong, kie-kang, pe-fan, hoaang-pĕ, kan-tsao, kin-tay* (7ᵍ,36); pulvériser; miel (3ᵍ,68); eau chaude.

Tr 39.2 *Bleed.* [Give :-] **nán pào shā săn** 南泡沙散 *Adenophora Powder*:

- *nan-pong-cha* = **nán pào shā** 南泡沙 Adenophora potaninii root (other spp. used similarly). Adenophora.
- *hoang-lien* = **huáng lián** 黃連（黄连）Coptis spp. rhizome. Goldthread.
- *jin-seng* = **rén shēn** 人參（人参）Panax ginseng root. Ginseng.
- *po-ho* = **bò hé** 薄荷 Mentha haplocalyx herb. Field mint.
- *tchuen-hiong* = **chuān xiōng** 川芎 Ligusticum chuanxiong rhizome. Sichuan lovage root.

- *kie-kang* = **jié gĕng** 桔梗 Platycodon grandiflorus root. Balloon flower.
- *pe-fan* = **bái fán** 白礬（白矾）Alum.
- *hoaang-pĕ* = **huáng băi** 黄柏（黄柏）Phellodendron spp. bark. Amur cork tree.
- *kan-tsao* = **gān căo** 甘草（甘艸）Glycyrrhiza spp. root. Licorice. Liquorice.
- *kin-tay* = **qīng dài** 青黛 Isatis indigotica leaf. Woad.

7.36g [of each].

Reduce to a powder.

- miel = **honey.**   *3.68g.*
- **hot water.**

§ **Fr 40.1** *Chou-tsao-pou-tong.*

Constipation, inappétence, plaintes; le bœuf se couche.

§ **Tr 40.1** *chū cǎo bù tōng*
出艸不通（出草不通）
grass exit blockage

Constipation, lack of appetite, groaning; the ox lies down.

Fr 40.2 Remède : *Tie-lao-san. - To-san-long, ty-kou-py, mou-tong, hoang-lien, ta-hoang, tien-tchou-hoang, fou-ling, tong-tchao, kië-kang, ou-oey-tsee, houei-hoa* (7^g,36); pulvériser.

Tr 40.2 Remedy :- ***dié láo sǎn*** 跌勞散（跌劳散） *Falling-Down Taxation Powder*:

- *to-san-long* = ***tǔ sàn lóng*** 土散龍（土散龙）Earthworm.
- *ty-kou-py* = ***dì gǔ pí*** 地骨皮 Lycium spp. root bark. Wolfberry.
- *mou-long* = ***mù tōng*** 木通 Akebia spp. stalk. Akebia.
- *hoang-lien* = ***huáng lián*** 黃連（黄连）Coptis spp. rhizome. Goldthread.
- *ta-hoang* = ***dà huáng*** 大黃（大黄）Rheum spp. root/rhizome. Rhubarb.
- *tien-tchou-hoang* = ***tiān zhú huáng*** 天竺黃（天竺黄）Tabasheer. Siliceous secretions of bamboo.
- *fou-ling* = ***fú líng*** 茯苓 Poria cocos. Poria. China root.
- *tong-tchao* = ***dōng zǎo*** 東棗（东枣）Zizyphus spinosa fruit. Sour jujube.

- *kië-kang* = **jié gěng** 桔梗 Platycodon grandiflorus root. Balloon flower.
- *ou-oey-tsee* = **wǔ wèi zǐ** 五味子 Schisandra spp. fruit. Five-flavour berry.
- *houei-hoa* = **huǐ huā** 檓花 Zanthoxylum bungeanum. pericarp. Sichuan pepper.

7.36g [of each].

Reduce to a powder.

§ **Fr 41.1**   Remède général pour la maladie appelé *ouen-y-ping* :

§ **Tr 41.1**   A general remedy for the disease known as ***wēn yì bìng*** 溫疫病（温疫病）*warm epidemic disease* :

Fr 41.2 *Sy-sin, ou-kia-py, tien-hoa* (racine), *ty-kou-py, houei-ing* (7ᵍ,36),   œuf (1), musc (0ᵍ,03).

Tr 41.2   [℞ :]

- *sy-sin* = ***xì xīn*** 細辛（细辛）Asarum spp. root/rhizome. Chinese wild ginger.
- *ou-kia-py* = ***wǔ jiā pí*** 五加皮 Eleutherococcus gracilistylus root bark. Acanthopanax.
- *tien-hoa* (racine) = ***tiān huā (fěn)*** 天花（粉）Trichosanthes kirilowii/rosthornii root. Chinese cucumber.
- *ty-kou-py* = ***dì gǔ pí*** 地骨皮 Lycium spp. root bark. Wolfberry.
- *houei-hiang* = ***huí xiāng*** 茴香 Foeniculum vulgare fruit. Fennel.

7.36g [of each].

- ***egg.***   *1*

- musc = ***musk.***   *0.03g [30mg].*

[Compare ℞ in **53.2**, **56.2** & **58.2** below.]

§ Fr 42.1	Ulcères :

§ Tr 42.1   Ulcers :

Fr 42.2 *Lieou-hoang* (2^g), *kou-kiao* (72^g), *san-lay* (36^g); pulvériser; faire huile et frotter.

Tr 42.2 [℞ :]

- *lieou-hoang* = **liú huáng** 硫黄（硫黄）Sulphur/Sulfur.   *2g.*

- *kou-kiao* = **kú qiáo** 苦蕎（苦荞）Fagopyrum tartaricum seed. Bitter buckwheat.   *72g.*

- *san-lay* = **sān lài** 三賴（三赖）Kaempferia galanga rhizome. Galangal.   *36g.*

                    Reduce to a powder.

- huile = **oil.**

Rub on.

§ **Fr 43.1**	Pour donner de la sueur :

§ **Tr 43.1**   To induce sweating :

Fr 43.2 *Ching-ma, tang-kouei, tchuen-hiong, kan-tsao, ma-hoang, cho-yo, jin-seng, tsee-kou-py, hiang-fou* (7ᵍ,36), eau.

Tr 43.2 [℞ :]

- *ching-ma* = **qǐng má** 苘麻 Abutilon theophrasti seed. Chingma abutilon. Chinese jute. Indian mallow.

- *tang-kouei* = **dāng guī** 當歸（当归）Angelica sinensis root. Chinese angelica.

- *tchuen-hiong* = **chuān xiōng** 川芎 Ligusticum chuanxiong rhizome. Sichuan lovage root.

- *kan-tsao* = **gān cǎo** 甘草（甘艸）Glycyrrhiza spp. root. Licorice. Liquorice.

- *ma-hoang* = **má huáng** 麻黃（麻黄）Ephedra spp. leaf/stem. Ephedra.

- *cho-yo* = **sháo yào** 芍藥（芍药）Paeonia spp. rubra root. Red peony root.

- *jin-seng* = **rén shēn** 人參（人参）Panax ginseng root. Ginseng.

- *tsee-kou-py* = **cì qiū pí** 刺楸皮 Kalopanax septemlobus bark. Kalopanax.

- *hiang-fou* = **xiāng fù** 香附 Cyperus rotundus rhizome. Nutgrass.

7.36g [of each].

- **water.**

§ **Fr 44.1**   Urine avec sang :

§ **Tr 44.1**   Blood in the urine :

Fr 44.2 *Hiong-hoang, tchou-cha, hai-kin-cha, ma-pien-tsao, pe-ye, tang-kouei, kan-tsao, ma-hoang, ou-kia-py* (4^g); *pulvériser; eau chaude.*

Tr 44.2 [℞ :]

- *hiong-hoang* = ***xióng huáng*** 雄黃（雄黄）Realgar. Ruby of arsenic.
- *tchou-cha* = ***zhū shā*** 朱砂 Cinnabar. Red mercury sulphide.
- *hai-kin-cha* = ***hǎi jīn shā*** 海金沙 Lygodium japonicum spores. Lygodium.
- *ma-pien-tsao* = ***mǎ biān cǎo*** 馬鞭艸（马鞭草）Verbena officinalis herb. European verbena.
- *pe-ye* = ***bǎi yè*** 柏葉（柏叶）Platycladus orientalis leaves. Chinese thuja.
- *tang-kouei* = ***dāng guī*** 當歸（当归）Angelica sinensis root. Chinese angelica.
- *kan-tsao* = ***gān cǎo*** 甘草（甘艸）Glycyrrhiza spp. root. Licorice. Liquorice.
- *ma-hoang* = ***má huáng*** 麻黃（麻黄）Ephedra spp. leaf/stem. Ephedra.
- *ou-kia-py* = ***wǔ jiā pí*** 五加皮 Eleutherococcus gracilistylus root bark. Acanthopanax.

4g [of each].

Reduce to a powder.

- ***hot water****.*

§ **Fr 45.1**	Toux :

§ **Tr 45.1**   Cough :

Fr 45.2 Feuilles de thé, miel (36^g), *hoa-kiao* (15^g), gingembre (15^g); faire bouillir.

Tr 45.2 [℞ :]

- Feuilles de thé = ***tea leaves.***

- miel = ***honey***.   *36g.*

- *hoa-kiao* = ***huā jiāo*** 花椒 Zanthoxylum spp. pericarp. Sichuan pepper.   *15g.*

- gingembre = ***ginger.***   *15g.*

- ***Boil.***

[Compare ℞ in **49.2** below.]

§ **Fr 46.1**   Vomissement de sang :

§ **Tr 46.1**   Vomiting blood :

Fr 46.2 *Chou-yn, ko-tsee, pe-tsee, jo-tchong-jong* (3ᵍ,68), eau chaude.

Tr 46.2 [℞ :]
- *chou-yn yu* = **shǔ yù** 薯蕷（薯蓣） Dioscorea opposita rhizome. Chinese yam.
- *ko-tsee* = **kǔ zǐ** 苦子 Brucea javanica fruit. Brucea.
- *pe-tsee* = **bái zhǐ** 白芷 Angelica dahurica root. Dahurican angelica.
- *jo-tchong-jong* = **ròu cōng róng** 肉蓯蓉（肉苁蓉） Cistanche deserticola herb. Desert broomrape.

3.68g [of each].

- **hot water.**

§ **Fr 47.1**   Selles mêlée de sang :

§ **Tr 47.1**   Stools mixed with blood :

Fr 47.2 Terre rouge dans de l'eau bouillie.

Tr 47.2 [℞ :]
- terre rouge = ***chì tiě kuàng*** 赤鐵礦（赤铁矿）Iron oxide mineral. Haematite/Hematite.
                          in
- ***boiling water.***

§ Fr 48.1	Oppression, sueur, naseaux froids :

§ Tr 48.1 Breathlessness, sweating, cold nostrils :

Fr 48.2 Graines des pêches avec graines de grenades (72^g chacune); faire bouillir.

Tr 48.2 [℞ :]
- graines des pêches = ***peach stones.***
- graines de grenades = ***pomegranate seeds.***

72g of each.

- ***Boil.***

§ Fr 49.1	Toux :

§ Tr 49.1   Cough :

Fr 49.2 Tabac (36^g), *teou-tsee* (36^g); faire bouillir.

Tr 49.2 [℞ :]
- tabac = **tobacco.**
- *teou-tsee* = ***tù xī*** 菟奚 Tussilago farfara flower. Colt's foot.

36g of each.

- ***Boil.***

[Compare ℞ in **45.2** above.]

§ Fr 50.1	Cou enflé :

§ Tr 50.1   Swollen neck :

Fr 50.2 *Han-choui-che, ty-yu-py, seng-ty, hoa-che, po-siao, che-yen* (36^g); faire bouillir.

Tr 50.2 [℞ :]

- *han-choui-che* = **hán shuǐ shí** 寒水石 Calcite. Calcium carbonate mineral.
- *ty-yu-py* = **dì yú pí** 地榆皮 Sanguisorba officinalis root bark. Burnet-bloodwort.
- *seng-ty* = **shēng dì** 生地 Rehmannia glutinosa root. Chinese foxglove.
- *hoa-che* = **huá shí** 滑石 Talcum.
- *po-siao* = **pǔ xiāo** 朴消 Glauber's salt. Mirabilite.
- *che-yen* = **shí yán** 石鹽 (石盐) Rock salt.

36g [of each].

- ***Boil.***

§ **Fr 51.1**   Ne peut ouvrir la bouche :

§ **Tr 51.1**   Unable to open the mouth :

Fr 51.2 Graines de légumes avec *ma-tsee* (250^g) ; .

Tr 51.2 [Give :]

- graines de légumes = ***cài zǐ*** 菜籽 Rapeseed.
                        with
- *ma-tsee* = ***má zǐ*** 麻滓 Sesame seed cake (residue remaining after extraction of oil).

                                        250g [of each].

§ **Fr 52.1**   Maladie *sin-hoang* :

§ **Tr 52.1**   *xīn huáng bìng*
                                  心黃病（心黄病）
                                  yellow heart malady :
                          [see above: **7.1** & compare ℞ in **7.2**]

Fr 51.2   *Pe-tsee, ta-hoang* (150ᵍ); faire bouillir.

Tr 52.2 [℞ :]

- *pe-tsee* = ***bái zhǐ*** 白芷 Angelica dahurica root. Dahurican angelica.
- *ta-hoang* = ***dà huáng*** 大黃（大黄）Rheum spp. root/rhizome. Rhubarb.

150g [of each].

- ***Boil.***

---

§ **Fr 53.1**   Autre maladie *ouen-y* :

---

§ **Tr 53.1**   Another [R for] malady ***wēn yì [bìng]*** 溫疫［病］（溫疫［病］）*warm epidemic [disease]* :

Fr 53.2   Donner *fou-ling* (4^g), *ta-hoang*, *tsang-pou* (72^g); poudre; eau chaude.

Tr 53.2   Give :-

- *fou-ling* = ***fú líng*** 茯苓 Poria cocos. Poria. China root.   *4g.*

- *ta-hoang* = ***dà huáng*** 大黃（大黃）Rheum spp. root/rhizome. Rhubarb.   *72g.*

- *tsang-pou* = ***chāng pú*** 菖蒲 Acorus calamus rhizome. Sweetflag.   *72g.*

                                                Reduce to a powder.

- ***hot water.***

[Compare R in **41.2** above, & **56.2** & **58.2** below.]

§ Fr 54.1	Autre, ulcère sur la langue :

§ Tr 54.1   Another [℞], [for] ulcer on the tongue :

Fr 54.2 *Tang-hiang* (4ᵍ), *mou-hiang* (4ᵍ), *che-ming* (0ᵍ,03), *ngay-sy-hiang* (0ᵍ,03), *hoang-pe* (11ᵍ), *hoang-lien* (11ᵍ), *ta-hoang* (11ᵍ), *yu-kin* (15ᵍ), *tsee-tsee* (15ᵍ); poudre; eau chaude.

Tr 54.2 [℞ :]

- *tang-hiang* = ***tán xiāng*** 檀香 Santalum album. Sandalwood.
  4g.

- *mou-hiang* = ***mù xiāng*** 木香 Aucklandia lappa root. Saussurea.
  4g.

- *che-ming* = ***xī míng*** 菥蓂 Thlaspi arvense seeds. Thlaspi.
  0.03g [30mg].

- *ngayn-sy-hiang* = ***ān xī xiāng*** 安息香 Styrax spp. resin. Benzoin.
  0.03g [30mg].

- *hoang-pe* = ***huáng bǎi*** 黄柏（黄柏）Phellodendron spp. bark. Amur cork tree.
  11g.

- *hoang-lien* = ***huáng lián*** 黄連（黄连）Coptis spp. rhizome. Goldthread.
  11g.

- *ta-hoang* = ***dà huáng*** 大黃（大黄）Rheum spp. root/rhizome. Rhubarb.
  11g.

- *yu-kin* = **yù jīn** 鬱金（郁金）Curcuma spp. root. *Inc.* turmeric. *15g.*

- *tsee-tsee* = **zhī zǐ** 梔子（栀子）Gardenia jasminoides fruit. Cape jasmine. *15g.*

Reduce to a powder.

- **hot water.**

[Compare ℞ in **64.2** below.]

---

§ Fr 55.1   Vomissement, diarrhée :

---

§ Tr 55.1   Vomiting, diarrhoea :

Fr 55.2 *Tchuen-yu-kin, hoan-tchong, pe-fan, kin-kuen-che, cha-jin, kiang-ko, hoa-che, ping-long-ken, chan-to-ken, kan-tsao, tsien-lieou, che-kao, kin-kiai, tsee-tsee, ta-hoang, mou-tong, hoang-lien* (7ᵍ,36); poudre (36ᵍ), eau chaude.

Tr 55.2 [℞ :]

- *tchuen-yu-kin* = **chuān yù jīn** 川鬱金（川郁金） Curcuma chuanyujin tuber. Curcuma.
- *hoan-tchong* = **guàn zhòng** 貫眾（贯众） Cyrtomium fortunei rhizome. Cyrtomium.
- *pe-fan* = **bái fán** 白礬（白矾） Alum.
- *kin-kuen-che* = **jīn zuàn shí** 金鑽石（金钻石） Corundum.
- *cha-jin* = **shā rén** 砂仁 Amomum spp. fruit. Grains-of-paradise.
- *kiang-ko* = **jiāng zhū** 江珠 Succinum. Amber.
- *hoa-che* = **huá shí** 滑石 Talcum.
- *ping-long-ken* = **bīng láng zhān** 檳榔鈷（槟榔鈷） Sargentodoxa cuneata stems. Sargentodoxa vine.
- *chan-to-ken* = **shān dòu gēn** 山豆根 Menispermum dauricum rhizome. Asiatic moonseed.
- *kan-tsao* = **gān cǎo** 甘草（甘艸） Glycyrrhiza spp. root. Licorice. Liquorice.
- *tsien-lieou* = **chēng liǔ** 檉柳（柽柳） Tamarix chinensis twig & leaf. Tamarisk.
- *che-kao* = **shí gāo** 石膏 Crystalline gypsum.
- *kin-kiai* = **jīn jié [gěng]** 津桔［梗］ Platycodon grandiflorus (southern variety) root. Balloon flower.

- *tsee-tsee* = **zhī zǐ** 栀子（栀子）Gardenia jasminoides fruit. Cape jasmine.
- *ta-hoang* = **dà huáng** 大黃（大黄）Rheum spp. root/rhizome. Rhubarb.
- *mou-tong* = **mù tōng** 木通 Akebia spp. stalk. Akebia.
- *hoang-lien* = **huáng lián** 黃連（黄连）Coptis spp. rhizome. Goldthread.

7.36g [of each].

Reduce to a powder.

[Give] 36g [of powder in] :

- ***hot water.***

§ **Fr 56.1**   Autre, *ouen-y.* -

§ **Tr 56.1**   Another [℞ for malady] ***wēn yì [bìng]*** 溫疫［病］(溫疫［病］) *warm epidemic [disease]* :-

Fr 56.2   *Che-tsang-pou, ko-ken, tan-tchou-ye, yu-kin, la-teou, tsang-chou* (11ᵍ,04), eau chaude.

Tr 56.2 [℞ :]
- *che-tsang-pou* = ***shí chāng pú*** 石菖蒲 Acorus tartarinowii rhizome. Grassleaf sweetflag.
- *ko-ken* = ***gé gēn*** 葛根 Pueraria spp. root. Kudzu vine.
- *tan-tchou-ye* = ***dàn zhú yè*** 淡竹葉 (淡竹叶) Lophaterum gracile stems & leaves. Lophaterum.
- *yu-kin* = ***yù jīn*** 鬱金 (郁金) Curcuma spp. root. *Inc.* turmeric.
- *la-teou* = ***lǜ dòu*** 綠豆 (绿豆) Phaseolus radiatus seed. Mung bean.
- *tsang-chou* = ***cháng chǔ*** 萇楚 (苌楚) Actinidia chinensis/rufa fruit. A type of kiwi fruit.

11.04g [of each].

- ***hot water.***

[Compare ℞ in **41.2** & **53.2** above, & **58.2** below.]

§ Fr 57.1	Inappétence, maigreur :

§ **Tr 57.1**   Lack of appetite, thinness :

Fr 57.2   Tabac, *teou-tsee, hoang-pe* (36^g); poudre; eau tiède.

Tr 57.2 [℞ :]
- Tabac = ***tobacco.***
- *teou-tsee* = ***tù xī*** 菟奚 Tussilago farfara flower. Colt's foot.
- *hoang-pe* = ***huáng bǎi*** 黃柏（黄柏）Phellodendron spp. bark. Amur cork tree.

36g [of each].

- ***lukewarm water.***

§ **Tr 58.1**   Another [℞ for malady] ***wēn yì [bìng]*** 溫疫［病］（温疫［病］）*warm epidemic [disease]* :-

Fr 58.2 *Tsang-chou, tchuen-hiong, tchuen-ou, tsao-ou, tang-kouei, kan-tsao, ho-siang, ty-long, fou-ling, pe-tchou, po-ho, kin-kiai, ta-houang, san-tsy, tchin-py, hiang-fou, ma-hoang, tsee-sou, cho-yo, tsiang-ko, hoa-che, hoang-tsien, kiai-y-san* (7ᵍ,20); poudre fine (36ᵍ) chaque fois.

Tr 58.2 [℞ :]

- *tsang-chou* = ***cháng chǔ*** 萇楚（苌楚）Actinidia chinensis/rufa fruit. A type of kiwi fruit.
- *tchuen-hiong* = ***chuān xiōng*** 川芎 Ligusticum chuanxiong rhizome. Sichuan lovage root.
- *tchuen-ou* = ***chuān wū*** 川烏（川乌）Aconitum carmichaelii main tuber. Aconite.
- *tsao-ou* = ***cǎo wū*** 草烏（草乌）Aconitum kusnezoffii prepared root. Wild aconite.
- *tang-kouei* = ***dāng guī*** 當歸（当归）Angelica sinensis root. Chinese angelica.
- *kan-tsao* = ***gān cǎo*** 甘草（甘艸）Glycyrrhiza spp. root. Licorice. Liquorice.
- *ho-siang* = ***huò xiāng*** 藿香 Agastache rugosa. Korean mint.
- *ty-long* = ***dì lóng*** 地龍（地龙）Earthworm.
- *fou-ling* = ***fú líng*** 茯苓 Poria cocos. Poria. China root.
- *pe-tchou* = ***bái chǒu*** 白丑 Pharbitis spp. seed. Morning glory.
- *po-ho* = ***bò hé*** 薄荷 Mentha haplocalyx herb. Field mint.
- *kin-kiai* = ***jīn jié [gěng]*** 津桔［梗］Platycodon grandiflorus (southern variety) root. Balloon flower.

- *ta-houang* = ***dà huáng*** 大黃（大黄）Rheum spp. root/rhizome. Rhubarb.
- *san-tsy* = ***sāng zhī*** 桑枝 Morus alba twigs. Mulberry.
- *tchin-py* = ***chén pí*** 陳皮（陈皮）Citrus reticulata aged peel. Tangerine.
- *hiang-fou* = ***xiāng fù*** 香附 Cyperus rotundus rhizome. Nutgrass.
- *ma-hoang* = ***má huáng*** 麻黃（麻黄）Ephedra spp. leaf/stem. Ephedra.
- *tsee-sou* = ***zǐ sū*** 紫蘇（紫苏）Perilla frutescens fruit. Perilla.
- *cho-yo* = ***sháo yào*** 芍藥(芍药) Paeonia spp. rubra root. Red peony root.
- *tsiang-ko* = ***xiāng gǎo [běn]*** 香藁［本］Ligusticum spp. rhizome. Chinese lovage.
- *hoa-che* = ***huá shí*** 滑石 Talcum.
- *hoang-tsien* = ***huáng qín*** 黃芩（黄芩）Scutellaria baicalensis root. Baical skullcap.
- *kiai-y-san* = ***jiē yī [téng] sǎn*** 結衣［藤］散（结衣［藤］散）Parabarium micranthum bark powder.

7.2g [of each].

Reduce to a fine powder.
[Dose:] 36g each time.

[Compare R in **41.2**, **53.2** & **56.2** above.]

---

§ Fr 59.1 Diarrhée continuelle :

---

§ Tr 59.1 Continual diarrhoea :

Fr 59.2 *Tchuen-hiong, kou-kiao, chan-yo, seng-ty, hoang-la* (11ᵍ,04), miel; faire bouillir.

Tr 59.2 [℞ :]

- *tchuen-hiong* = **chuān xiōng** 川芎 Ligusticum chuanxiong rhizome. Sichuan lovage root.
- *kou-kiao* = **kú qiáo** 苦蕎(苦荞) Fagopyrum tartaricum seed. Bitter buckwheat.
- *chan-yo* = **shān yào** 山藥(山药) Dioscorea opposita rhizome. Chinese yam.
- *seng-ty* = **shēng dì** 生地 Rehmannia glutinosa root. Chinese foxglove.
- *hoang-la* = **huáng là** 黃蠟(黄蜡) Beeswax.

11.04g [of each].

- miel = **honey.**

- **Boil.**

---

§ **Fr 60.1** Maladie des chaleurs :

---

§ **Tr 60.1** Heat disorder :

Fr 60.2 *Fou-ling, ho-po, ho-siang, tsang-chou, tchan-py, tsin-py, jou-kouei, jin-seng, ping-lang* (3ᵍ,68); poudre *ou-mey* (7ᵍ), eau.

Tr 60.2 [℞ :]

- *fou-ling* = **fú líng** 茯苓 Poria cocos. Poria. China root.
- *ho-po* = **hòu pò** 厚朴 Magnolia officinalis bark. Magnolia.
- *ho-siang* = **huò xiāng** 藿香 Agastache rugosa. Korean mint.
- *tsang-chou* = **cháng chǔ** 萇楚（苌楚） Actinidia chinensis/rufa fruit. A type of kiwi fruit.
- *tchan-py* = **chén pí** 陳皮（陈皮） Citrus reticulata aged peel. Tangerine.
- *tsin-py* = **qīng pí** 青皮 Citrus reticulata green peel. Tangerine.
- *jou-kouei* = **ròu guì** 肉桂 Cinnamomum cassia inner bark. Saigon cinnamon.
- *jin-seng* = **rén shēn** 人參（人参） Panax ginseng root. Ginseng.
- *ping-lang* = **bīng láng** 檳榔（槟榔） Areca catechu nut. Betel.

3.68g [of each].

- poudre *ou-mey* = **wū méi sǎn** 烏梅散（乌梅散） *Mume Powder (Black Plum Powder)* * 7g.

- **water.**

*[Note :-]

---

*This was (& still is) a well-known preparation. Although not given by Dabry, its formula is equal weights of :-

- **wū méi** 烏梅（乌梅）Mume fruit. Black plum.
- **huáng lián** 黃連（黄连）Coptis spp. rhizome. Goldthread.
- **jiāng húang** 薑黃（姜黄）Curcuma spp. root. Turmeric.
- **hē zǐ** 訶子（诃子）Terminalia chebula fruit. Chebula.

To these, may be added :-

- **gān shì** 乾柿（干柿）Diospyrus kaki dried calyx. Persimmon.

§ Fr 61.1 L'animal remue constamment, mucosités coulant par la bouche ;

§ Tr 61.1 The animal moves about constantly, mucus flowing fom its mouth :

Fr 61.2 *Hiang-fou, tchin-py, kan-tsao, san-tsee, nan-sin, jo-kouei, tsay-hou, ta-fou-py, ping-lang* (7^g,36); poudre; avec *tang-kouei* (36^g); faire bouillir.

Tr 61.2 [℞ :]

- *hiang-fou* = **xiāng fù** 香附 Cyperus rotundus rhizome. Nutgrass.
- *tchin-py* = **chén pí** 陳皮（陈皮）Citrus reticulata aged peel. Tangerine.
- *kan-tsao* = **gān cǎo** 甘草（甘艸）Glycyrrhiza spp. root. Licorice. Liquorice.
- *san-tsee* = **sāng zhī** 桑枝 Morus alba twigs. Mulberry.
- *nan-sin* = **nán xīng** 南星 Arisaema erubescens prepared rhizome. Jack-in-the-pulpit.
- *jo-kouei* = **ròu guì** 肉桂 Cinnamomum cassia inner bark. Saigon cinnamon.
- *tsay-hou* = **chái hú** 柴胡 Bupleurum spp. root. Hare's ear.
- *ta-fou-py* = **dà fù pí** 大腹皮 Areca catechu husk. Betel nut husk.
- *ping-lang* = **bīng láng** 檳榔（槟榔）Areca catechu nut. Betel.

7.36g [of each].

Reduce to a powder.

Together with :-

- *tang-kouei* = **dāng guī** 當歸（当归）Angelica sinensis root. Chinese angelica.   *36g.*

- **Boil.**

§ **Fr 62.1**   Empoisonnement miasmatique :

§ **Tr 62.1**   Miasmatic poisoning :

Fr 62.2 *Pe-cho, seng-ty, jo-kouei, kiu-kiai, tchuen-hiong, tang-kouei, tsay-hou, fang-fong, jin-seng, sien-mao-ken, kan-tsao* (7^g,36); poudre et eau chaude.

Tr 62.2 [℞ :]

- *pe-cho* = ***bai sháo*** 白藥（白药） Paeonia spp. alba root. White peony root.

- *seng-ty* = ***shēng dì*** 生地 Rehmannia glutinosa root. Chinese foxglove.

- *jo-kouei* = ***ròu guì*** 肉桂 Cinnamomum cassia inner bark. Saigon cinnamon.

- *ki#n-kiai* = ***jīn jié [gěng]*** 津桔［梗］ Platycodon grandiflorus (southern variety) root. Balloon flower.
  [Less likely: ***jiǔ jié*** 九節（九节） Psychotria rubra leaves, roots & twigs. Wild coffee.]

- *tchuen-hiong* = ***chuān xiōng*** 川芎 Ligusticum chuanxiong rhizome. Sichuan lovage root.

- *tang-kouei* = ***dāng guī*** 當歸（当归） Angelica sinensis root. Chinese angelica.

- *tsay-hou* = ***chái hú*** 柴胡 Bupleurum spp. root. Hare's ear.

- *fang-fong* = ***fáng fēng*** 防風（防风） Saposhnikovia divaricata root. Saposhnikovia.

- *jin-seng* = ***rén shēn*** 人參（人参） Panax ginseng root. Ginseng.

- *sien-mao-ken* = ***xiān máo gēn*** 仙茅根 Curculigo orchoides rhizome. Golden eye-grass.

- *kan-tsao* = **gān cǎo** 甘草（甘艸）Glycyrrhiza spp. root. Licorice. Liquorice.

7.36g [of each].

Reduce to a powder.

- **hot water.**

§ **Fr 63.1**   [Empoisonnement miasmatique]
                  Autre remède :

§ **Tr 63.1**   [Miasmatic poisoning]
                  Another remedy :

Fr 63.2 *Tchou-cha* (7ᵍ,36), *jou-hiang* (7ᵍ,36), *ping-pien* (4ᵍ), *che-hiang* (2ᵍ), *po-siao* (15ᵍ), *tsee-tsee* (15ᵍ), *kou-hoang-lien* (15ᵍ), *kin-hoa* (12ᵍ), *kin-kiai* (15ᵍ), *hoa-che* (15ᵍ), *tsiang-ho* (15ᵍ), *tou-ho* (15ᵍ), *fang-fong* (20ᵍ), *tchuen-hiong* (20ᵍ), *kan-tsao* (36ᵍ), *ou-oey-tsee* (11ᵍ), *po-ho* (15ᵍ); poudre (36ᵍ), chaque fois, un peu d'eau chaude.

Tr 63.2 [℞ :]

- *tchou-cha* = **zhū shā** 朱砂 Cinnabar. Red mercury sulphide.
                                                    7.36g.

- *jou-hiang* = **rù xiāng** 乳香 Olibanum. Frankincense.   *7.36g.*

- *ping-pien* = **bīng piàn** 冰片 Borneol.   *4g.*

- *che-hiang* = **shè xiāng** 麝香 Moschus. Musk.   *2g.*

- *po-siao* = **pǔ xiāo** 朴消 Glauber's salt. Mirabilite.   *15g.*

- *tsee-tsee* = **zhī zǐ** 栀子（梔子） Gardenia jasminoides fruit.
  Cape jasmine.   *15g.*

- *kou-hoang-lien* = **chǎo huáng lián** 炒黃連（炒黄连）Coptis
  spp. dry-fried rhizome. Goldthread.   *15g.*

- *kin-hoa* = **jīn guā** 金瓜 Cucurbita pepo fruit. Field pumpkin.
  12g.

- *kin-kiai* = **jīn jié [gěng]** 津桔［梗］ Platycodon grandiflorus (southern variety) root. Balloon flower. *15g.*

- *hoa-che* = **huá shí** 滑石 Talcum. *15g.*

- *tsiang-ho* = **qiāng huó** 羌活 Notopterygium spp. rhizome or root. Notopterygium. *15g.*

- *tou-ho* = **dú huó** 獨活（独活）Angelica pubescens root. Pubescent angelica. *15g.*

- *fang-fong* = **fáng fēng** 防風（防风）Saposhnikovia divaricata root. Saposhnikovia. *20g.*

- *tchuen-hiong* = **chuān xiōng** 川芎 Ligusticum chuanxiong rhizome. Sichuan lovage root. *20g.*

- *kan-tsao* = **gān cǎo** 甘草（甘艸）Glycyrrhiza spp. root. Licorice. Liquorice. *36g.*

- *ou-oey-tsee* = **wǔ wèi zǐ** 五味子 Schisandra spp. fruit. Five-flavour berry. *11g.*

- *po-ho* = **bò hé** 薄荷 Mentha haplocalyx herb. Field mint.
  15g.

Reduce to a fine powder.
[Dose:] 36g each time

- *in a little **hot water**.*

§ **Fr 64.1**   Ulcère sur la langue :

§ **Tr 64.1**   Ulcer on the tongue :

Fr 64.2 *Hoa-che, po-siao, kin-tay, pe-fan, hiong-pê, chan-to-ken* (7^g,36); pulvériser; miel, et mettre sur la langue.

Tr 64.2 [℞ :]

- *hoa-che* = **huá shí** 滑石 Talcum.
- *po-siao* = **pǔ xiāo** 朴消 Glauber's salt. Mirabilite.
- *kin-tay* = **qīng dài** 青黛 Indigo.
- *pe-fan* = **bái fán** 白礬 (白矾) Alum.
- *hiong*-pê* = **xiāng bǎi** 香柏 Platycladus orientalis leaves. Chinese thuja.   *[a probable typo: *hiong* = *hiang*.]
- *chan-to-ken* = **shān dòu gēn** 山豆根 Menispermum dauricum rhizome. Asiatic moonseed.

7.36g [of each].

Reduce to a powder.

[*Add* :-]

- miel = **honey.**

Apply to the tongue.

[Compare ℞ in **54.1** above.]

§ Fr 65.1	Ophthalmie :

§ Tr 65.1   Ophthalmia :

Fr 65.2 *Fang-fong, kin-kiai, hoa-che, hoang-lien, tsee-tsee, kin-hoa* (11ᵍ); poudre; eau tiède.

Tr 65.2 [℞ :]

- *fang-fong* = **fáng fēng** 防風（防风）Saposhnikovia divaricata root. Saposhnikovia.
- *kin-kiai* = **jīn jié [gěng]** 津桔［梗］Platycodon grandiflorus (southern variety) root. Balloon flower.
- *hoa-che* = **huá shí** 滑石 Talcum.
- *hoang-lien* = **huáng lián** 黃連（黄连）Coptis spp. rhizome. Goldthread.
- *tsee-tsee* = **zhī zǐ** 栀子（栀子）Gardenia jasminoides fruit. Cape jasmine.
- *kin-hoa* = **jīn guā** 金瓜 Cucurbita pepo fruit. Field pumpkin.

11g [of each].

Reduce to a powder.

- **lukewarm water.**

§ **Fr 66.1**   Blessures du garrot et en deçà du garrot :

§ **Tr 66.1**   Injuries to the withers & below the withers :

Fr 66.2 Coton torréfié et pulvérisé avec *hiang-yeou,* et frotter.

Tr 66.2 [℞ :]
- ***cotton,*** torrefied & reduced to a powder.
               with
- *hiang-yeou* = ***xiāng yóu*** 香油 Sesame oil.

Rub on.

§ Fr 67.1	Ulcère à l'anus :

§ Tr 67.1   Anal ulcer :

Fr 67.2   Coquilles d'œufs, *tie-tsee* (feuilles), *tse-hoa* (feuilles); faire bouillir; frotter avec de l'huile. — *Ming-fan, hiong-hoang, hoang-lien, lien-kiao, tchuen-chan-kia* (7ᵍ,36), *kin-fen* (7ᵍ,36); pulvériser; eau chaude; donner à prendre.

Tr 67.2 [℞ :]

[Externally :-]

- coquilles d'œufs = ***eggshells.***
- *tie-tsee* (feuilles) = ***tiĕ zĭ*** 鐵子（铁子） Myrsine africana leaves. African boxwood.
- *tse-hoa* (feuilles) = ***shí huā*** 石花 Davallia tenuifolia leaves. Rabbit foot fern.

- ***Boil.***

- *Rub in with **oil.***

Give by mouth :-
- *ming-fan* = ***ming fán*** 明礬（明矾） Alum.
- *hiong-hoang* = ***xióng huáng*** 雄黃（雄黄） Realgar. Ruby of arsenic.
- *hoang-lien* = ***huáng lián*** 黃連（黄连） Coptis spp. rhizome. Goldthread.
- *lien-kiao* = ***lián qiáo*** 連翹（连翘） Forsythia suspensa fruit. Forsythia.

- *tchuen-chan-kia* = **chuān shān jiǎ** 穿山甲 Pangolin scales.
- *kin-fen* = **qīng fěn** 輕粉（轻粉） Calomel. Mercury chloride mineral.

7.36g [of each].

Reduce to a powder.

- **hot water.**

[End]

_____

INDEX OF SUBJECTS
According to Section Nº

32. Cow's seasonal disease.
33. Dropsical lameness disease.
34. Taxation disease.
35. Stomach reflex flushing disease.
36. Lung taxation disease.
37. Kidney & intestine disease.
38. Bladder vacuity disease.
39. Liver yellow swelling.
40. Grass exit blockage.
41. Warm epidemic disease.
42. Ulcers.
43. To induce sweating.
44. Bloody urine.
45. Cough.
46. Vomiting blood.
47. Bloody stools.
48. Breathlessness, sweating & cold nostrils.
49. Cough.
50. Swollen neck.
51. Unable to open mouth.
52. Yellow heart malady.
53. Warm epidemic disease.
54. Lingual ulcer.
55. Vomiting & diarhoea.
56. Warm epidemic disease.
57. Lack of appetite & thinness.
58. Warm epidemic disease.
59. Continual diarrhoea.
60. Heat disorder.
61. Restlessness & nasal mucus.
62. Miasmatic poisoning.
63. Miasmatic poisoning.
64. Lingual ulcer.
65. Ophthalmia.
66. Withers injuries.
67. Anal ulcer.

SOME IMPORTANT CHINESE WORKS ON LIVESTOCK MEDICINE PUBLISHED BEFORE 1863 *

* For those books devoted especially to equine medicine, see:
Practical equine diagnosis & treatment in late Qing imperial China.
Lessell, C.B. (2019). Suthsaexe, England: Samphire Press.

221-207 B.C.   Qin Dynasty.

❖ *Jiu yuan lu* (Animal husbandry & veterinary laws).

206 B.C.-220 A.D.   Han Dynasty.

❖ *Xiang liu chu* (Exterior of the six kinds of domestic animals). Published in 38 volumes.

265-581 A.D.   Jin to Southern-Northern Dynasties.

❖ *Qi min yao shu* (Basic techniques for farmers). Written by Jia Sie Xie around 533-544.

581-618 A.D.   Sui Dynasty.

❖ *Zhi ma niu tuo luo deng jing* (The classics on the treatment of diseases in horses, cattle, camel & mule).

960-1127 A.D.   Song Dynasty.

❖ *Fan mu zuan yan fang* (Tested prescriptions of nomad origin). Written by Wang Yu, a veterinarian, around 1086-1110. A collection of 57 veterinary prescriptions as well as animal acupuncture techniques.

1368-1644 A.D.   Ming Dynasty.

❖ **1608.** *Yuan Heng liao ma ji fu niu tuo jing* (Yuan & Heng's classics on the treatment of equine diseases, with cattle & camel diseases attached). Published in 1608, it was written by Yu Ben Yuan and Yu Ben Heng. It covers basic theory, diagnosis, acupuncture, therapeutics, and castration. A revised edition was published in 1736 (see below).

❖ **1633.** *Xin bian ji cheng ma yi fang niu yi fang* (The new collection of prescriptions for horses & cattle). It was written by two Koreans, Zhao Jun and Jin Shi Heng, prefaced by a Chinese, Fang Shi Liang, and published in Chinese in 1633.

From 1644 A.D.   Qing Dynasty.

❖ **1736.** *Yuan Heng liao ma ji fu niu tuo jing*, originally issued in 1608 (see above), was published in a revised form in 1736 by Li Yu Shu. It is still the most popular text in use today. However, the compositions of many of Dabry's compound medicines differ, to varying degrees, from those given in *Yuan Heng*. See also *Ma niu tuo jing da quan* below (1785).

❖ **1758.** *Chuan ya shou yi fang* (Compiled veterinary formulas). Published in 1758, & written by Zhao Xue Min, it contains the most popuar herbal formulas for treating horses, other mammals, birds, etc.

❖ **1785.** *Ma niu tuo jing da quan* (The complete collection of diseases of horses, cattle & camels). An annotated version of *Yuan Heng liao ma ji fu niu tuo jing* (see1608 above) published by Guo Huai Xi in 1785.

❖ **1800.** *Yang geng ji* (A collection on management of farm cattle). Written by Fu Shufeng, it includes diagnosis & prescriptions.

❖ **c. 1800.** *Bao du ji* (Treatise on calf diseases). Author unknown.

❖ **1815.** *Niu yi jin jian* (Reference on treating cattle diseases). Published in two parts, it is of unknown authorship.

中国晚清实用牛羊医学

牛羊草药手册

从一八六三年的原始
法文和中文文本转录和翻译

Dr. Colin B. Lessell

二零二零